A GREEN GUIDE TO YOUR

Natural Pregnancy
and Birth

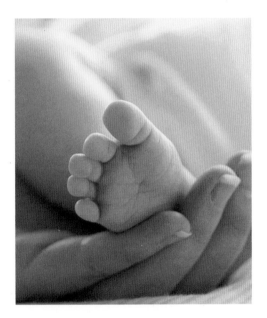

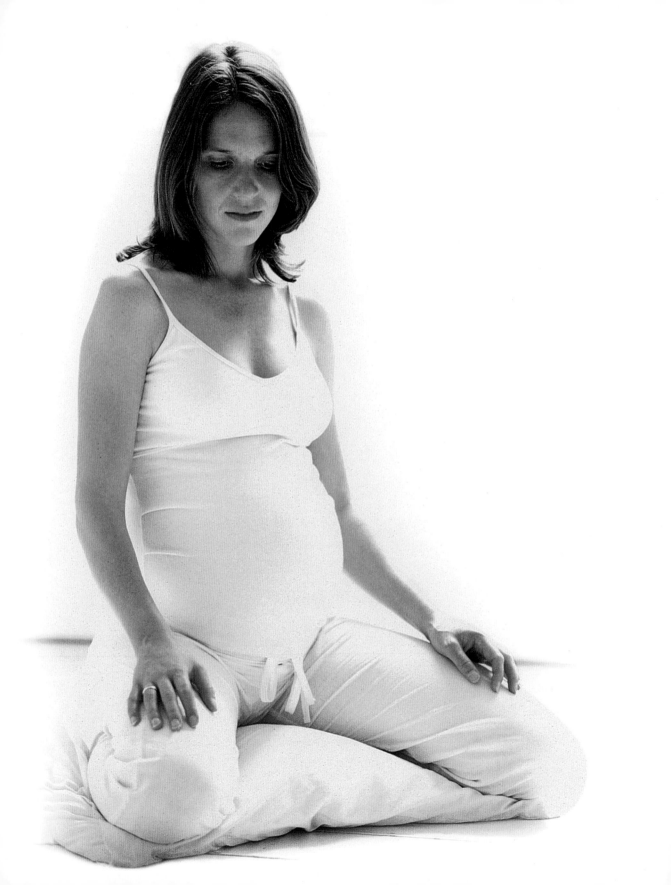

A GREEN GUIDE TO YOUR

Natural Pregnancy
and Birth

the kind way for you, your baby, and the environment

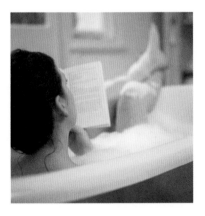

claire gillman

CICO BOOKS
LONDON NEW YORK

This book is dedicated to the woman who carried me so well for nine months—my lovely mum, Eileen May Gillman.

Published in 2010 by CICO Books
an imprint of Ryland Peters & Small
519 Broadway, 5th Floor, New York, NY 10012

www.cicobooks.com

10 9 8 7 6 5 4 3 2

A CIP catalog record for this book is available from the Library of Congress.

ISBN-13: 978-1-907030-79-6

Printed in China

Copy editors: Katie Hardwicke and Eleanor van Zandt
Designer: Barbara Zuñiga

Please note that the advice in this book is not to be considered as a substitute for medical advice from your family doctor or any other qualified medical practitioner. If you treat yourself with natural medicines, such as herbs, you should always inform your doctor, because these can be very powerful and can interact with prescribed and over-the-counter medications.

Contents

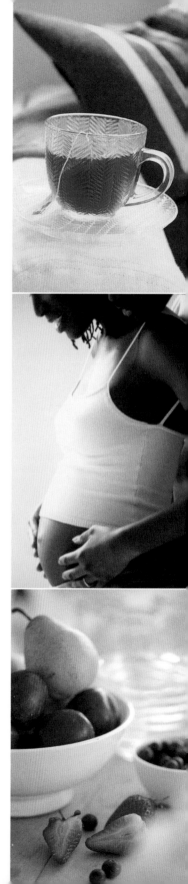

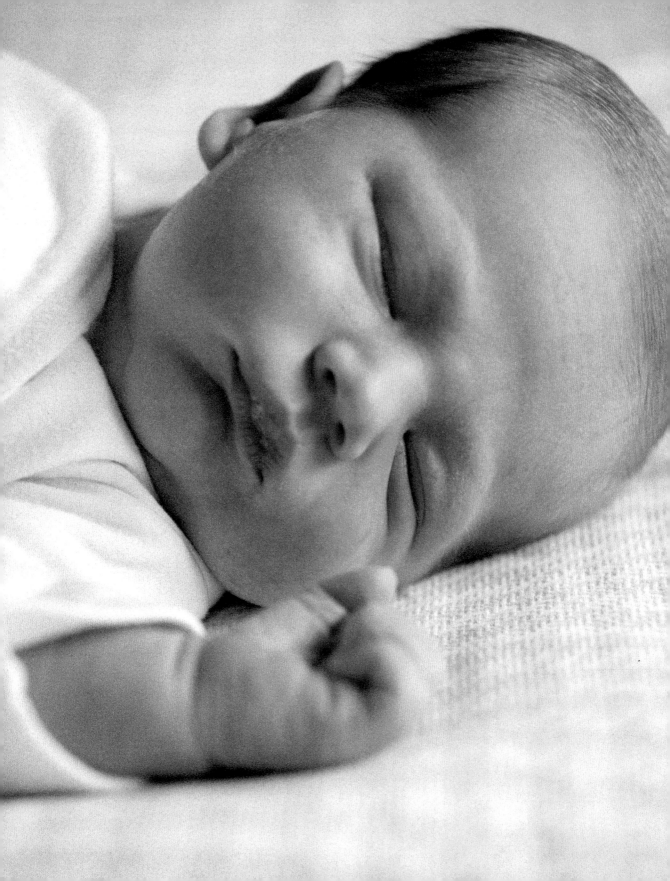

Introduction

Finding out that you are expecting a baby is such monumental news. It can be joyous, shocking, overwhelming, but is always of huge significance and probably the biggest life-changing event you will ever experience. It seems to me that there is never a better time than when you are pregnant to embrace a greener approach to life, your body, and our planet.

By investigating and seeking natural products, noninvasive treatments, and drug-free approaches to pregnancy and birth, you are actively taking steps to ensure a happy and healthy conclusion to your pregnancy—namely, a healthy and hearty baby.

The aim of this book is to help you to enjoy your pregnancy in the most natural way possible and in a manner that fits in with your particular beliefs and lifestyle. It is written with all women in mind, regardless of how much or how little you want to adopt a natural approach. Some of you will be keen to espouse most of the advice contained in these pages; others will be happy to cherry-pick the suggestions that best resonate with themselves. Either way is fine.

Of course, what we now call a natural pregnancy and active birth used to be the norm. It was only during the twentieth century, with the ascendance of obstetricians, that it was decided that pregnancy and childbirth needed greater monitoring and more medical intervention. Although still less than 1 percent of American babies and 2.7 percent of British babies are born at home, these figures are on the increase, and there appears to be a seachange in women's attitudes to how their pregnancy and birth are handled. More and more women are keen to take back ownership and responsibility for their prenatal health and to be less passive in giving birth to their babies.

That is not to say that modern medicine does not have its place, and this book is certainly not anti-medical. Indeed, thanks to advances in conventional medicines and obstetric care, premature babies born as young as 24 weeks now stand a very good chance of survival. And in an emergency or an out-of-the-ordinary pregnancy, the medical treatment you will receive is often essential and potentially lifesaving.

My point is that the vast majority of pregnancies and births are not emergencies. They are low-risk, and because of this, both mother and baby can benefit from a more natural approach. Your body is perfectly capable of sustaining a blooming and joyful pregnancy and supporting the healthy growth and development of your unborn child. By being prepared and informed about your birth options, you can approach labor with a sense of control and confidence, too.

The information in this book aims to give you choice and the confidence to take control over your body. Most pregnant women are reluctant to pop a pill that might have unexpected side effects, but there is no need to suffer during pregnancy. The chapter on Remedies and Therapies guides you through a host of natural therapies that are suitable and safe during pregnancy, and in Health and Well-being you will find complementary therapies and natural self-help remedies that can see you comfortably through many of the common pregnancy ailments.

You can prepare yourself emotionally for the life-changing events of pregnancy, birth, and looking after your newborn baby, too. Your pregnancy is a perfect time in which to build a relationship between yourself and the baby in your womb, who is aware of and sensitive to your moods and feelings. This forms a loving foundation on which you can build your future relationship with your son or daughter.

The chapter on Healthy Living contains practical, commonsense advice on how to protect yourself and baby from unnecessary exposure to harmful chemicals and pollutants in the home environment, as well as the workplace. In addition, there's general advice, such as how to eat healthily and how to ensure your physical and emotional well-being, so that you can enjoy your pregnancy to the full.

This book aims to give you useful information about your pre-conception and prenatal care, and preparation for labor, birth, and the early postnatal period. It is wonderful that you are informing yourself on these issues so that you can make confident decisions. However, I also believe that moms-to-be instinctively know what is right for them and their unborn child; and, as a starting point in all pregnancy matters, you should trust your intuition.

The contents of this book are by no means exhaustive, but there should be more than enough practical suggestions here to guide you through a natural, comfortable, and rewarding pregnancy that leads to a happy and healthy baby and lays the foundation for a green and healthy future for your new family.

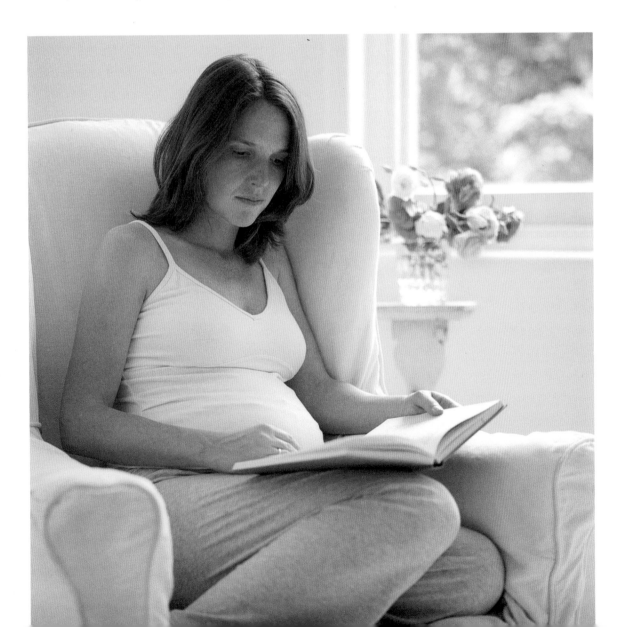

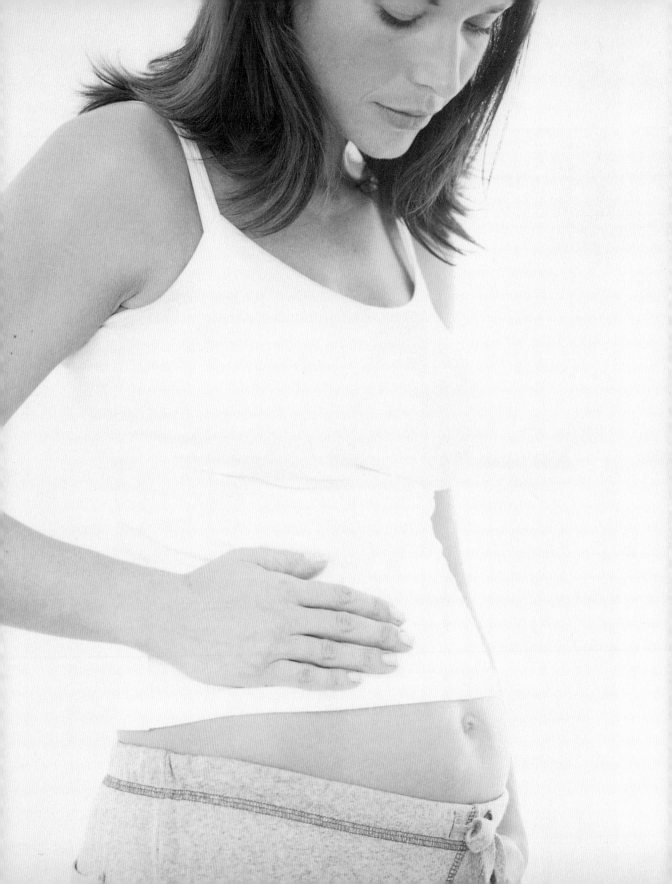

Your Pregnancy Milestones

The week-by-week calendar in this chapter (see pages 14–19) charts the many changes that you can expect in your body and emotions as you progress through each trimester of your pregnancy. Alongside, you will find a guide to how your baby begins to develop and grow inside. Some of the changes to yourself, especially the physical ones, are very obvious; but you may be less sensible to other, more subtle alterations. Meanwhile, your baby's milestones are reached on an almost weekly basis and are quite astonishingly remarkable.

The illustrated monthly timeline (see pages 12–13) takes you step-by-step from the moment of conception to the birth of your new baby, so that you can see at a glance how you might look, plus what might be happening in your life at that particular stage of your pregnancy. It's not only reassuring and comforting but also strangely exciting to be able to see what comes next—so enjoy!

Pregnancy Timetable

This month-by-month calendar pictorially charts the progress in one woman's pregnancy. You may notice many of the same changes in your body and emotions as you move toward your due date.

The 40 weeks of pregnancy are calculated from the first day of your last menstrual period. After conception, your baby actually takes only 38 weeks to develop. So, when using these milestones (and the ones on the following pages), bear in mind that there is some leeway in how far along you are in your pregnancy, depending on whether or not your menstrual cycle is an exact 28 days. However, this chart will give you a general idea of the stage of growth that your baby is at.

Pregnancy Timeline

Month 1
Whether you've taken a home pregnancy test or been to your doctor to confirm the news, it will take a little while for it to sink in. However, it's surprising how many women know or suspect they've conceived before a urine test confirms the news.

Month 2
Although you look the same, you may be feeling very different. It's entirely up to you when you decide to share your news with friends and loved ones; but this stage, when it's just a secret between you and your partner, can feel very special and intimate.

Month 3
The physical discomforts of early pregnancy should be wearing off, but you'll need a proper maternity bra about now. You might want to start thinking about telling your employer and enrolling for prenatal exercise classes.

Month 4
As you start to feel much better, now's the time to get excited. You may need to get some natural-fiber maternity clothes, too, as your ordinary clothes will probably become too tight at this stage.

Month 5
Many women report a sense of well-being at this stage and are often described as "radiant," due to improvements in skin and hair. You should be enjoying the thrill of feeling your baby move around now.

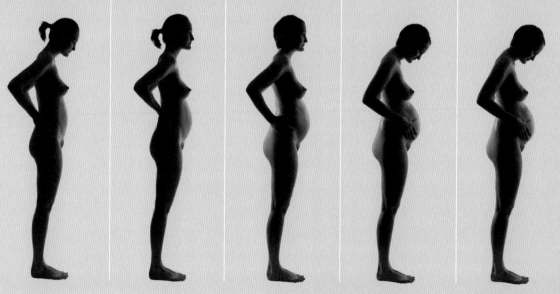

Conception

You are most fertile about 14 days before your period is due. At this time, a ripe egg is released from one of your ovaries. It travels down the Fallopian tube; then, if not fertilized, it passes out of the vagina along with the womb lining, as your next period.

However, if a sperm successfully enters the egg during its journey down the tube, fertilization takes place and the egg and sperm fuse together to form a single cell. It continues to divide as it travels down the Fallopian tube. On about the fourth day after fertilization, the egg reaches the womb. By now, it is a ball of about 100 cells, and for the next few days, it floats freely in the womb. After about three weeks, the fertilized egg attaches itself to the soft lining of the womb. The egg sends projections into the lining of the womb that eventually join up with the mother's blood vessels and form the elementary beginnings of the placenta.

greenfile

Remember: every pregnancy is unique, and your experiences may differ greatly from those of your friends or textbook cases.

Month 6
This is the month when you start to pile on the pounds, and most women appear visibly pregnant by now. Pay attention to your posture, and practice gentle exercise, together with relaxation and breathing techniques.

Month 7
You're probably starting to feel large and clumsy, and are possibly growing more forgetful. Don't forget to let your employer know, in writing, when you intend to stop work. You're entering the homestretch now.

Month 8
As your body prepares for the birth, you will need as much rest as possible, so take naps if you are not sleeping as well as usual. Now is the time to start attending prenatal classes, if you haven't already done so, and buying baby essentials —what fun!

Month 9
The "nesting instinct" is often strong, so don't be surprised if you find yourself cleaning out closets and tidying the house. Buy your nursing bras and check that everything is ready for the baby. By now, you are probably impatient to give birth, and the wait is almost over.

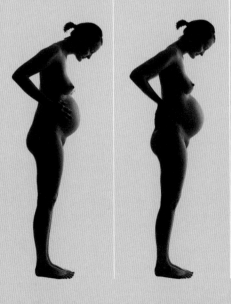
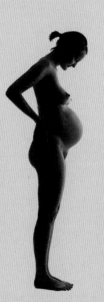
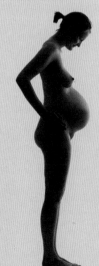

First Trimester

Your Baby's Milestones

Weeks 1–3
Six or seven days after fertilization, the developing cell mass, known as a blastocyst, becomes embedded in the uterus, where it multiplies fast.

Weeks 4–6
By week 4, your baby is about $\frac{1}{16}$ in (2 mm) long and weighs less than $\frac{1}{28}$ oz (1 g). Body tissues are starting to form, and at week 5, the heart has started to develop.

Week 6
Now an embryo, your baby's heart is beating at about 180 beats per minute. It has eyelids, ears, and the beginnings of hands and feet. The head and the curve of the spine can be distinguished.

Week 7
It is starting to move its body, arms, and legs, although you cannot feel the movements yet. The nervous system, lungs, kidney, and liver are starting to develop.

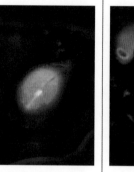
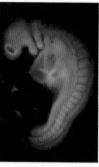
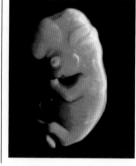

Your Pregnancy Timeline

First Trimester
Up to Week 12
In the early weeks of pregnancy you may experience:
- Enlarged, tender breasts, which may tingle slightly
- A strange metallic taste in your mouth
- Feeling rather emotional and easily upset because of hormonal changes
- A frequent need to pass water
- Nausea and perhaps vomiting at any time of the day, even though it's called "morning sickness"
- Tiredness
- Feeling faint and dizzy
- A strong dislike of certain tastes, especially tea, coffee, alcohol, toothpaste, and cigarettes, but a craving for others
- An increase in normal vaginal discharge

Week 8

At this stage, your baby has evolved into a fetus that is about 1 in (2.5 cm) in length. It can open and close its mouth, and ears are beginning to form. Its brain is developing rapidly.

Week 9

Your baby is now 1½ in (4 cm) long, and its brain has quadrupled in size in the past four weeks.

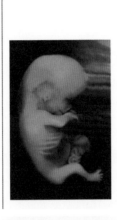

Week 10

Your baby now looks like a miniature human being, and all its organs are fully formed. The amniotic sac has formed, and your baby is moving around more, because its nervous system is more mature (but you won't feel it yet).

Week 11

Now about 2 in (5 cm) long, your baby has a fully formed face, and its liver and kidneys are beginning to function.

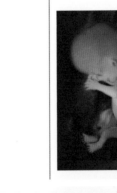

Week 12

Remarkably, your baby is now fully formed, although it's only 2½ in (6 cm) long. Its nails and hair are starting to grow, it has all 32 teeth buds, and it is starting to suck. His or her sex organs have now formed.

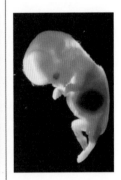

Week 12

You may find that:

• You feel less nauseous

• You don't need to pass water quite so often

• You get constipated as bowel movements tend to become sluggish during pregnancy

• You cease to feel the cold because the volume of blood circulating in your body increases

Second Trimester
Your Baby's Timeline

Week 13
Your baby's body is growing rapidly and he is supported by the placenta.

Week 14
Your baby can discern sound and light and responds to touch. He will swallow amniotic fluid and excrete it. The limbs are fully formed.

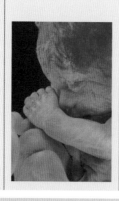

Week 15
Your baby is moving more vigorously now, and the bones are hardening. As he becomes more active, you may start to notice movement—often a light, fluttering sensation—particularly when you're resting.

Week 16
Your baby now has fingerprints and is covered in a downy hair all over the body, known as lanugo. Nipples appear, and the back, which has been curved, straightens.

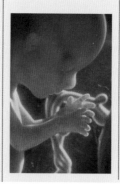

Week 17
Your baby is about 7 in (18 cm) long and weighs about 6 oz (170 g). He has facial expressions, and eyelashes and eyebrows are developing.

Your Pregnancy Timeline

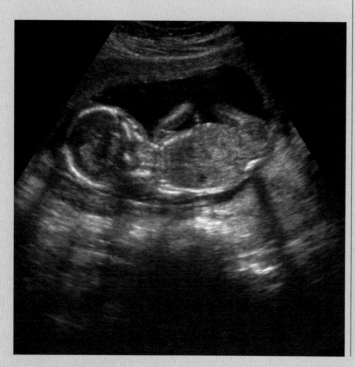

Week 16
You may find that:
• You're feeling much better
• Your nipples and the areola may darken, and a faint line, called the linea nigra, may appear down the center of your stomach—this fades after the birth
• You may no longer be able to fit into your ordinary clothes

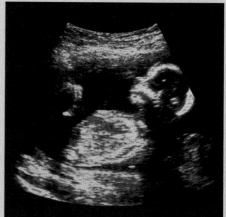

Weeks 18–20

Your baby may start to suck his thumb. The spinal cord is thickening, and by the end of this period, he will have reached roughly half his length at birth. Hair is growing on the head and the rate of growth starts to slow.

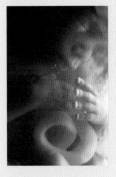

Weeks 21–23

Your baby has taste buds, and the ears are fully formed so he can hear and respond to music, sounds, and your speaking/singing/crying, etc. Your baby can also grip with the hands and may occasionally grasp the umbilical cord.

Week 24

He can open the eyes and identify voices. The heartbeat may now be discernible by fetoscope and will usually range between 120 and 160 beats per minute. The skin is translucent, and blood vessels can be clearly seen through it.

Weeks 25–26

The baby has wakeful and sleeping periods. He is covered in vernix—a white, waxy substance that nourishes and waterproofs the skin.

Week 27

This sees the start of another growth spurt, and your baby will start to put on weight.

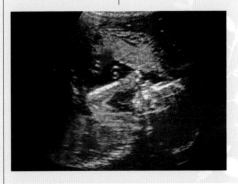

Week 20

You may find that:
• You feel great, even radiant, as you pass into the middle months of the pregnancy
• Your breasts may produce small amounts of colostrum, which is a clear, thin liquid
• Physical reactions may include bleeding gums and vaginal discharge
• Your joints and ligaments have relaxed, so you are more prone to back trouble and aches and pains
• You may get patches of pigmentation on your face and body—these will fade after the birth
• Your nails split and break more easily

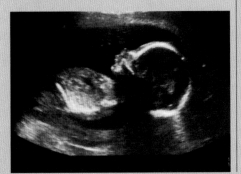

Week 24

You may find that:
• Your bump is growing rapidly
• You look a little puffy, as your body retains more water
• You sweat more, as you feel the heat
• You have a sudden weight gain

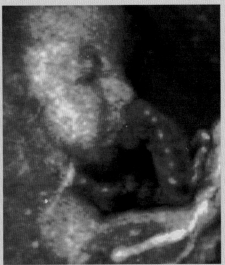

Third Trimester

Your Baby's Timeline

Week 28

If born now, although not fully matured, your baby would have a good chance of survival. Your baby's eyes are beginning to be able to focus, and if it's a boy, his testes have now descended into the groin.

Week 29

Your baby is now around 13 in (33 cm) long. The lungs have developed alveoli and are also producing a wetting agent, known as surfactant, to assist breathing at birth.

Week 30

Expect lots of movement now, because your baby has increased muscle tone.

Week 31

Your baby has been gaining weight at a rate of about 8 oz (250 g) a week. As fat deposits are laid down, his skin begins to smooth out and become pink, rather than red.

Weeks 32–33

Fingernails are fully grown (but not toenails) and the face has plumped out. Although your baby appears as you would expect to see him at birth, body systems are still maturing.

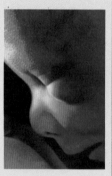

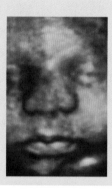

Your Pregnancy Timeline

Week 28

You may find that:
- You get shortness of breath, heartburn, indigestion, and cramps
- Stretch marks may appear on your stomach
- The veins on your breasts may become more pronounced
- You may put weight on your buttocks and thighs as well as your stomach
- You are having vivid and possibly frightening dreams. This is quite common and nothing to worry about. The dreams are not portentous but a product of your disturbed sleep

Week 32

You may find that:
- The pressure on your internal organs makes you breathless and need to pass urine frequently. You may find that you leak a little urine when you cough, sneeze, laugh, or run
- Your navel may have flattened or popped out
- You may be experiencing sleeping problems
- The base of your ribcage may be sore as the womb presses up under it
- You may experience discomfort in the pelvic region as the joints expand, ready for the birth

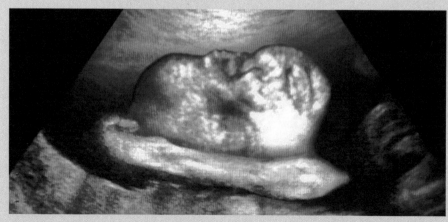

Weeks 34–35

The immune system is still developing, and your baby continues to receive your antibodies. However, the brain and nervous system are now fully developed. Your baby is about 14 in (36 cm) in length and weighs about 4 lb (2 kg). As your baby becomes more cramped in the space, he may start to move less.

Week 36

Meconium, a thick, green liquid consisting of dead cells and secretions from the liver and bowel, is beginning to form in the intestines (this will be your baby's first bowel movement). If your baby were born now, he should be mature enough to survive without too much difficulty.

Week 37

Your baby is rehearsing how to breathe, suck, and swallow. All of the sense organs are formed and he is ready for life outside of your womb. The baby has lost most of the lanugo and vernix that covered his body.

Week 38

Your baby is ready to be born. He is about 18–20 in (46–50 cm) long and weighs on average 6–9 lb (2.7–4 kg). There is very little room inside the uterus, and he has to curl up tightly. The head has now descended into the lower part of your pelvis, ready for birth.

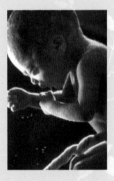

Week 36

You may find that:
• Some of the more unpleasant symptoms, such as breathlessness, heartburn, and indigestion, lessen as the baby's head drops into the pelvis
• You pass water a great deal
• You're tired and irritable
• You're apprehensive about the birth but want the pregnancy to be over
• The "nesting instinct" is strong. You have bursts of energy during which you clear out closets and prepare the home

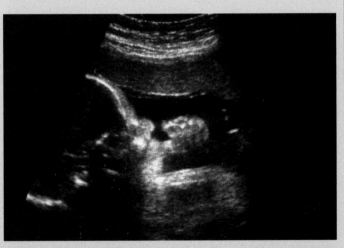

Week 40

You may find that:
• You have pins and needles in your legs
• You can't move around very easily
• Your lower abdomen feels drawn and heavy
• You experience Braxton Hicks contractions (also known as false labor)
• You lose a little weight or your weight gain tails off. This is a sign that the baby is full term

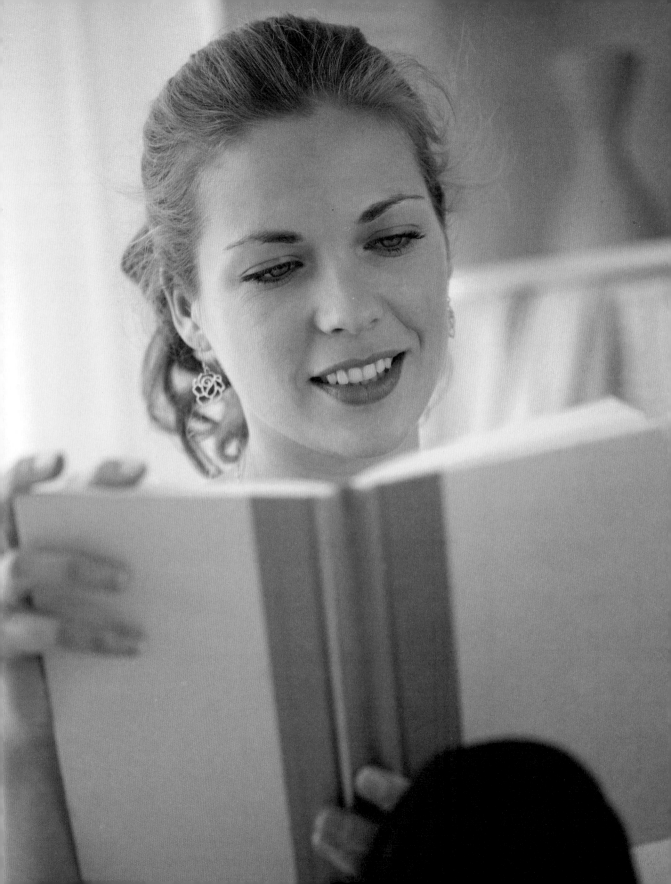

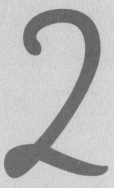
A Healthy Start

Discovering that you are pregnant is an exciting moment. However, as with any major life event, once the news has settled in, you can sometimes experience a mixture of emotions. This is perfectly natural. While in Western society, we place a great deal of emphasis on the obvious physical changes of pregnancy (see the illustrated monthly timeline on pages 12–13), in Eastern philosophy, it is equally important that you pay attention to your emotional and spiritual well-being (see page 32) and that you learn to listen intuitively to your body and its changes (see page 31).

In holistic circles, you hear people speak of the twelve months of pregnancy. Although it is commonly accepted that the physical growth of the baby takes only nine months, many consider the few months before conception to be as important as the nine-month term during which the fetus grows inside the womb. This is because, with good pre-conception preparation, your baby will get the best start it can toward a healthy life (see page 22).

So this chapter is devoted to making sure that you nurture yourself throughout the "twelve months" of pregnancy, keeping yourself healthy and well (see page 26), keeping your relationship strong (see page 34), and keeping yourself relaxed and stress free (see page 36).

Pregnancy is a wonderful time, despite the discomforts that are sometimes associated with it, and it offers a glorious opportunity for you to plan and think about the sort of parent(s) you might like to be.

Pre-conception Health

It is one of life's bitter ironies that some couples, having spent years worrying about contraception, then find it difficult to conceive when they eventually decide to have a baby.

In fact, for conception to take place successfully, you need a good foundation. You both need to be as fit and healthy as possible before trying to conceive if you are to:

- optimize the chances of conceiving
- reduce the risk of miscarriage
- improve the probability of carrying a pregnancy to full term
- increase the likelihood of delivering a healthy baby

In particular, the three-to-six-month period prior to conception plays a vital role in your baby's future, both physically and intellectually, and so it is important that both partners start preparing for a pregnancy at least three months before you want to conceive.

Lifestyle Changes

It is now known that health and lifestyle affect the fertility of both parents. If you have a pressurized job and lead a hectic social life, you may need to make a few adjustments.

It is recommended that both partners give up alcohol, smoking, and recreational drugs some months before trying to conceive. Street drugs, in particular marijuana, are known to reduce sperm production significantly, and the effects can take a considerable time to wear off. Tobacco affects the motility (active movement) of the sperm, while alcohol increases the number of dead and deformed sperm. Not only does this reduce your chances of conception, but it also increases the risks of miscarriage, should you be lucky enough to conceive, because an egg fertilized by a damaged sperm is more likely to be rejected by your body.

Obviously, the effects on the fetus from alcohol and tobacco consumption are well documented, but it is less well known that smoking reduces female fertility—a study by the National Institute of Environmental Health showed that female nonsmokers were more than three times more likely to conceive than smokers. Moreover, it is believed that alcohol inhibits the passage of the egg from the ovary to the womb, again adversely affecting female fertility.

The best advice is to give up drinking and smoking completely; but if this is too much of a tall order for you, at least cut down on your consumption, with a view to eventually giving up if possible (see pages 52 and 72).

Reducing Stress Levels

If you are stressed in your work or simply a naturally tense person, you may experience difficulty in getting pregnant. In women stress is thought to interfere with ovulation, while in men stress hormones inhibit sperm production.

In extreme cases, you may decide that it's worth changing your job, depending on how much your work is affecting your health. Usually, it is enough to invest time in learning techniques for stress management, in slowing down the pace of your lifestyle, and/or in using complementary therapies, such as aromatherapy massage or herbal remedies, to relax (see pages 106 and 112).

greenfile

Neroli, rose, and sandalwood essential oils can help to calm and relax. Essential oils, such as chamomile, lavender, and geranium, are good if you're feeling irritable and tense.

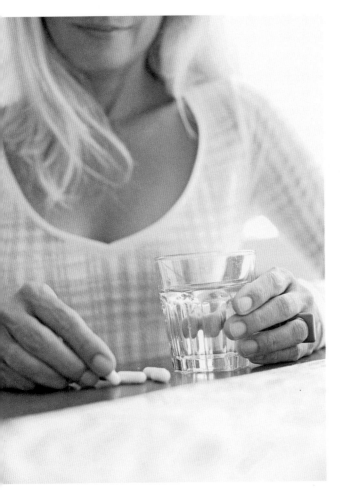

WEIGHT

You will conceive more readily and be less likely to suffer problems, such as high blood pressure, during pregnancy if you are within the normal weight range for your height.

Good Nutrition

Both prospective parents need a nutritious diet to produce healthy sperm and eggs, which in turn will produce a healthy fetus. Make an effort to include as much fresh fruit and vegetables, and meat and fish, in your diet as possible, plus plenty of wholegrain breads and cereals.

Vitamins and minerals are particularly important at this time, so if you find it difficult to eat a nutrient-rich diet, you should consider taking a multivitamin and mineral supplement (see page 58).

One of the key nutrients of paramount importance to women hoping to get pregnant is folic acid. A lack of folic acid in the diet can increase the risk of having a baby with spina bifida or other neural tube defects. So you should increase your intake of this important nutrient at least three months before you try to conceive and continue well into the pregnancy (for the first trimester at least). For natural sources of folic acid see page 44, and for supplements, see page 58.

Contraception

If you use hormone-based contraception, such as the Pill, most doctors recommend that you switch to a barrier method for about three months before trying to conceive. This allows your natural fertility cycle to reestablish itself—although this can take up to a year—and vitamin and mineral levels to return to normal. While you are on the Pill, the amounts of folic acid, vitamins C and E, and zinc in your blood are reduced, while iron and copper levels are raised. There's no direct evidence that this harms a developing fetus, but it may affect fertility. If you are fitted with an intrauterine contraceptive device (IUD or coil), have this removed at least a month before you plan to conceive.

Indeed, if it is taking you longer than you had hoped or expected to conceive, the pressure of trying to get pregnant can, in itself, be stressful. Try not to be disappointed if you don't see immediate results. As a generalization, nearly half of all couples trying to conceive are successful within six months, another 35 percent take up to a year, and the remaining 15 percent take longer and may need medical intervention. However, your doctor is unlikely to take any action with regard to infertility investigations unless you have been trying to conceive for at least a year and, in some cases, eighteen months.

So, although it may sound trite to say so, try not to be tense about getting pregnant. The more uptight you get each month that goes by, the harder it will be for you to conceive.

A Healthy Start   23

Medical Conditions

Symptomless genitourinary infections can impede conception and increase the risk of miscarriage and premature labor. Chlamydia is a common infection that often goes undetected, yet it can adversely affect your newborn baby, so it's worth getting yourself tested.

You should also let your doctor know that you are planning to conceive, so that s/he can monitor any prescription drugs s/he might normally prescribe. For example, antibiotics and certain asthma treatments can affect both male and female fertility, and you should always speak to the pharmacist before buying over-the-counter drugs during the three months prior to trying to conceive.

Finally, for women who have never had German measles (rubella) and who are uncertain about their vaccinations, it is important to ask your doctor for a blood test to check your immunity. If you contract rubella during pregnancy, it can damage your unborn child and cause serious birth defects. If you have no immunity, it is well worth getting the vaccination, but make sure you do so at least three months before trying to conceive.

> *greenfile*
>
> **False unicorn root (*Chamaelirium luteum*) is recommended for both men and women planning to conceive, because it strengthens and tones the reproductive system. It is available in capsule or tincture form, and the root or liquid extract can also be taken in a tea.**

Age

A woman is at the peak of her fertility in her mid-twenties. Thereafter, her fertility starts to decrease, and the decline is particularly acute after the age of 35. A man's fertility levels, on the other hand, stay pretty constant until he reaches his early fifties; and, biologically speaking, men are perfectly capable of fathering a child well into their eighties.

Timing

Make love as often as you like without getting too hung up on whether or not it's the right stage of your

---

BEFORE YOU CONCEIVE

Both you and your partner should:
- Give up smoking and recreational drugs
- Give up alcohol
- Eat a healthy, nutritious diet
- Reduce stress
- Check for genitourinary infections
- Monitor prescription drug use
- Take regular exercise, but not at excessive levels

You should:
- Stop using contraceptives
- Take extra folic acid (see page 23)
- Check immunity to rubella
- Avoid X-rays

YOUR PARTNER
The testes need to be several degrees cooler than body temperature because sperm production takes place at 89°F (32°C)—normal body temperature is 98.6°F (37°C).

He should:
- Wear loose fitting underwear and trousers
- Avoid sitting for long periods or crossing legs closely
- Avoid hot baths and electric blankets
- Turn the heating down
- Seek advice if he is in a hazardous occupation, such as working with radiation (for example, dentists and X-ray technicians) or using chemicals at work (for example, farmers or dry cleaners)

cycle. There is actually a three- or four-day period in the middle of your cycle (an egg is released from the ovary about 12–16 days before the next expected period, and this is your most fertile time) during which time you could conceive, so you don't have to leap on each other at the exact moment of ovulation.

Making love according to temperatures and calendars can, in itself, be stressful, and is certainly a turnoff. If you make love regularly three or so times a week, you will be doing enough to make conception likely to happen.

A Pre-conception Visit

A checkup is not necessary for everyone, but you should see your doctor if there is anything you want to discuss or if you have a chronic health problem that needs treatment. A visit can be useful in recognizing factors that might affect the timing or your decision to become pregnant, particularly in the case of women with significant health problems, such as diabetes, epilepsy, and congenital heart disease, and for couples with genetic risk factors.

A pre-conception appointment will provide:
- Risk assessment based on your medical histories, nutritional state, and personal/social issues
- Assessment of genetic concerns, with possible referral for genetic testing or counseling before pregnancy
- Immunization checks and updates
- Risk of Hepatitis B assessment
- Laboratory testing, if you have concerns about HIV, for example
- Contraception advice

greenfile

Although you can buy over-the-counter ovulation test kits, if you know your body well, you can detect your time of ovulation naturally: fluid from the vagina becomes thinner and wetter at this time, which is a good indication of ovulation.

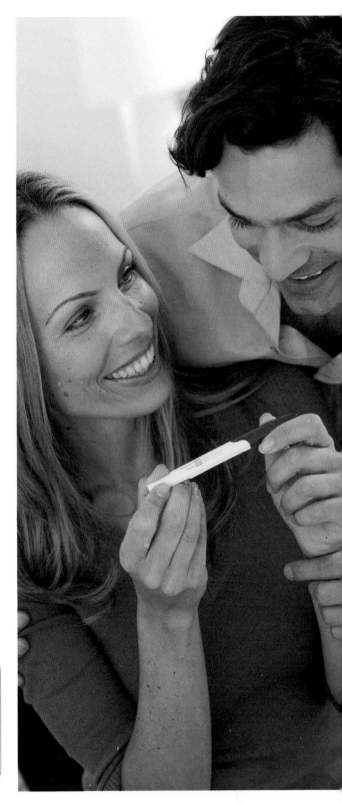

Taking Care of Yourself

At any stage of life, your health should always be an important consideration, but it is likely that you will be more conscious about keeping healthy during your pregnancy than at any other time.

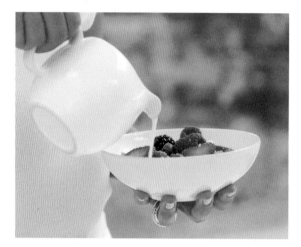

In part, that's because you know that if you fall ill, you may not be able to take the medications that you would normally resort to. However, it is also because you want to give your baby the very best start in life—and staying healthy is integral to that goal.

From a more selfish perspective, research shows that healthier mothers have shorter labors and recover faster after the birth. So, not only is staying healthy during pregnancy important for your unborn child's development, it's in your best interests, too!

Moreover, a healthy pregnancy lays the foundation of health to support you through your baby's early years. Obviously, a well-nourished, healthy mother is better able to cope with the stresses of early parenthood than one who is unhealthy.

So, how do you maintain good health throughout your pregnancy? The answer is not as complex as you might think. With a combination of nutritious eating and smart lifestyle choices, you are giving yourself the very best chance to stay healthy throughout your nine-month term.

Nutritious Eating

The following chapter (see page 42) is devoted to giving you the necessary nutritional information to make sure that your baby gets everything that it needs to grow and develop healthily and to keep you in optimum health.

However, it's worth pointing out here that, even when you are eating the right foods, there are still more ways that you can help yourself to stay healthy. For example, it's better for your digestive system to eat four to six small meals per day rather than three big ones. This is due to the fact that your stomach is being compressed by your growing baby and cannot hold as much food as it might normally.

So even if you're eating nutritiously, by eating little and often, you are helping your digestive system to remain healthy. This simple solution can help you to avoid one of pregnancy's most common ailments—heartburn (see page 122).

By the same token, you can reduce the likelihood of heartburn if you stay away from foods that you find hard to digest. These foods are, of course, peculiar to the individual, and you will know what yours are, but heartburn is more of a problem in pregnancy because your small and large intestines wrap around the uterus, so digestion takes longer than usual.

greenfile

To aid good digestion and to keep your body hydrated, you should drink at least eight glasses of liquid each day, preferably in the form of water, milk, unsweetened fruit juices, and fruit, herbal, or green tea.

Boosting Your Immunity

During pregnancy, your natural immunity is slightly lowered (in order to prevent your body rejecting the developing baby), which means that you will find you are more susceptible to illnesses, such as recurrent coughs and colds, fatigue, and bacterial, viral, or fungal infections.

There are a number of factors that can cause you to have a weakened immune system. For example, stress and anxiety depress the immune system, as does inadequate rest. A poor diet also deprives the body of the nutrients necessary to maintain a healthy immune system. Less well known is the fact that long-term use of antibiotics can cause impairment of the immune system.

You can help to boost your immune system by avoiding the above triggers and by eating foods rich in vitamins A, C, and E, zinc, and selenium (see pages 44–47 for natural food sources). These nutrients enhance your immune system and help the production of specialized white blood cells, which are mobilized to attack when a pathogen invades the body.

Complementary therapies, such as acupuncture, aromatherapy, and herbal remedies, can also be beneficial in supporting your body's immunity (see pages 101–117).

Pregnancy Exercise

A great way to stay healthy during your pregnancy is to maintain your fitness levels with safe, gentle exercise.

According to the American Congress of Obstetricians and Gynecologists (ACOG), regular exercise can:

- Ease backaches, constipation, bloating, and swelling
- Help to prevent or treat gestational diabetes
- Increase your energy
- Improve your mood
- Improve your posture
- Promote muscle tone, strength, and endurance
- Help you to sleep better
- Improve your ability to cope with the pain of labor
- Make it easier for your to get back in shape after the birth

However, you must be fairly sensible about exercising during pregnancy. Most forms of exercise are safe; but if you're new to exercise, choose a gentle, low-impact sport, such as swimming, walking, prenatal aerobics, aqua aerobics, yoga, or pilates.

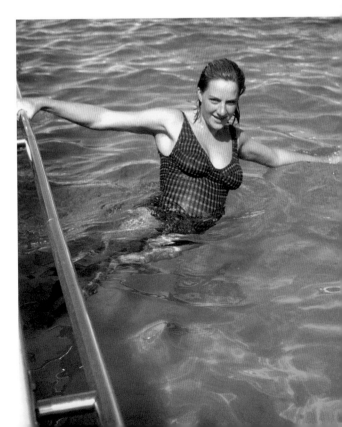

baby by flooding his body with the stress hormone cortisol, which can increase the rate of his heartbeat and raise his blood pressure. At the same time, stress can cause your body to suffer muscle cramps and increased heart rate, among other problems.

So make a concerted effort to slow your life down, to focus your attention on you and your baby, and to relax. You will find a number of recommended relaxation techniques later in this chapter (see page 36), but it is also useful to make a special space for yourself at this time—one where you can feel safe and secure and in which you can take refuge from life's daily stresses.

Why not set aside a room or an area of your bedroom where you can seek sanctuary. Light the special space with your favorite candles. Surround yourself with the scents that relax you—fragrant potpourri, incense, aromatherapy oils, scented candles, or fragrant bubble baths.

And finally, music is a subtle yet powerful way to affect your mood. You can use music to release mental energy and to relax tension in your body. Whatever your particular favorite, whether it's uplifting rock or atmospheric spiritual chants, find something that helps you to unwind and beat the stress of everyday life.

If you are already a regular sportswoman, it should be safe to continue with your chosen activity, although it is worth discussing this with your health practitioner first. Naturally, contact or extreme sports should be avoided. If your sport involves a risk of falling—for example, horse riding or waterskiing—you might be best advised to wait until after the birth to resume your activities.

Your new shape and body mass, coupled with the fact that the ligaments throughout your body are relaxed and joints are less stable, means that you should take care not to push yourself excessively or beyond what feels comfortable when exercising during pregnancy.

Beating Stress

In our modern age, it is almost impossible to avoid stress altogether. However, when you are pregnant, it is important to minimize your exposure to stressful factors as much as possible if you and your growing baby are to remain healthy. Stress not only adversely affects your own body and health; it also affects the

If you don't have family and friends living close by who are able to give you a helping hand, why not consider some professional help. A doula (see page 150) is a woman who offers emotional, mental, and physical support to mothers during pregnancy, childbirth, and the first weeks after the birth.

WARNING Research suggests that intensive exercise raises the mother's core body temperature and causes vasoconstriction (narrowed blood vessels), which reduces blood flow and thus oxygen supply to the uterus, and a raised fetal heart rate. Limit any strenuous exercise to 15 minutes maximum, and make sure the activity is supervised.

Changing Pace

It's very easy to push yourself too hard when you're pregnant. Like most women, you are probably used to juggling 101 different tasks and responsibilities at the same time. If you've always been an active, busy person and/or a hardworking professional, you're probably used to pushing yourself to get everything done before you collapse at the end of the day. And the odds are that you'll continue this pattern into your pregnancy. Most of the time, we manage to cope with this juggling act, but if you continually overextend yourself, especially during pregnancy, you will end up burning out.

You must be kind to yourself at this stage in your life. It is important during your pregnancy to listen to your body; to take time to rest or sleep when you feel tired; to stop overextending yourself. Instead, you need to draw your strength around you in order to stay healthy and to bring a healthy baby into the world. If this means accepting help from others, against all your instincts, then so be it. It is not a sign of weakness. On the contrary, it is a sign that you are listening to your body and to your woman's wisdom.

WOMEN'S WISDOM

Women's intuition is legendary, albeit often the butt of men's jokes, but now is a good time to tune in to your own intuitive knowledge. You may instinctively know what's right for you and your baby during pregnancy and labor. You may dream about your baby and feel that you know him before he's born. Your psychic skills may come to the fore, and you may be more aware of what's happening to family and loved ones through this sixth sense. Don't be afraid of this women's wisdom. It is there to help you, to allow you to be more comfortable with who you really are, and to assist you in tuning in to your body's own language.

Listen to Your Body

We would all benefit from listening to our bodies more closely at all stages of our lives, but pregnancy is the ideal time to start becoming more aware of what's happening in your body, because you are undergoing such dramatic physical and emotional transformations.

This is not merely about growing to accept and hopefully like your new shape. It's about thinking about your self-perception as your social role changes from individual woman to mother. It's about tuning in to your heightened physical and emotional sensations.

This is a unique time in your life, when you can allow yourself the time to immerse yourself in the language of your body. It is also perhaps the only time when other women are apt to speak about their bodies so openly; and as you share your experiences regarding the physical and emotional changes you are undergoing, so you become more comfortable and confident about listening to your own body and trusting the messages you receive.

Basic Signals

Perhaps the most obvious place to start is by paying attention to the most basic signals that your body will be giving out on a daily basis: namely, hunger, thirst, fatigue, and toilet necessities. Sounds pretty rudimentary doesn't it? But how often have you ignored the urge to go to the restroom, instead waiting for a more convenient time or putting it off until you can't wait any longer? In fact, if you do this repeatedly, you are in danger of getting a urinary tract infection, which is common during pregnancy.

Similarly, do you eat when you are hungry, or do you wait until the prescribed mealtimes? Worse still, do you try to curb your appetite because you fear putting on too much weight while pregnant? Listening to your body is so important at this time, and especially regarding food.

Signals that you are hungry should be obeyed. That's not an excuse to snack on candy and cookies. However, your body may require several smaller meals or snacks that are easier to digest, rather than eating three large meals a day.

Some signals need to be heard and interpreted. For example, if you have a craving for something sweet, your body may need more energy. Don't be tempted to ignore your body's signals and to override your feelings of fatigue by taking in coffee, chocolate, or sugar. That is a short-term and shortsighted solution. You'd be better recognizing your body's message that you need more energy and taking in some complex carbohydrates, such as nuts, cereal bars, or crackers with cheese, or eating protein-rich snacks, such as hard cheese or a tub of low-fat yogurt. Combining the two (a yogurt with cereal or nuts), will provide you with more lasting energy.

Signals that you may interpret as feeling a bit miserable or under the weather, such as feeling weepy, faint, irritable, cold or clammy, and headachy, could in fact mean that your blood sugar levels are too low and you need a square meal.

You'll soon find that your intuition rarely, if ever, lets you down. The more you recognize and respond to your body's signals, the better you will feel.

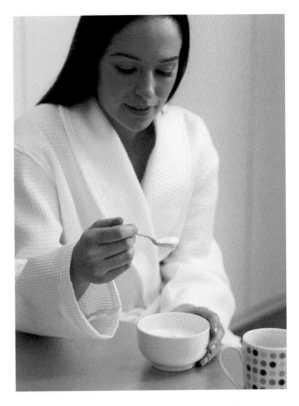

Emotional Well-being

No matter how amazing and, in some cases, longed for, a newly discovered pregnancy is, the truth remains that such news is rarely met with unconditional joy. Even when a pregnancy is planned, you are almost certain to experience a mixture of emotions when you discover for the first time that you are expecting a baby.

Even as you rejoice at the revelation, a small part of you may be overwhelmed by the magnitude of the news. A feeling of, "Oh my goodness, what have we done?" may accompany, or quickly follow, the initial euphoria—along with (in most cases) the weighty realization that there is no going back.

It is perfectly natural to have these doubts, because this is, after all, a life-changing event. For most women, though, anxieties over the impending changes in their bodies and lifestyle, or about whether this is the right time to have a baby, are simply lingering doubts in the back of the mind while they slowly take in the news.

Disbelief is another widespread reaction to a positive test. It's not uncommon for a woman to do several tests, all with positive results, and still believe that there's been a mistake or that her period will start soon.

Mood Changes

As your hormones run amok through your body, early pregnancy may become an emotional rollercoaster, as it is for many women. You may experience sudden changes in mood, you may find yourself very sensitive and tearful, or you may become rather self-absorbed and inward looking. All these reactions are very common, if a little bewildering. But if these emotional changes are slightly baffling to you, they are a downright mystery to the man in your life.

Hopefully, talking honestly and openly about your feelings and expectations with one another will give you a greater intimacy and will help him to feel an integral part of this time of wonder, rather than a mere observer.

Male Reactions

For most men, who don't have the physical reality of a missed period or early symptoms, pregnancy news is even more unreal. After all, you look no different.

Although, in the case of a planned pregnancy, the man is usually as delighted as the woman, he too will probably experience some feelings of apprehension. Although his body is not going to change, if he is committed to his new family, his lifestyle will undoubtedly alter.

He may be conscious and concerned about the unfamiliar responsibility of fatherhood. In many cases, men are profoundly affected by the pressure of knowing that they will have to provide for their family—perhaps only briefly, in cases where the mother returns to work, yet sometimes indefinitely. Some men feel able to meet the financial needs of a family but wonder about how they will cope with the emotional responsibilities of raising a child. An expectant dad may experience mixed emotions about the pregnancy itself as he becomes increasingly concerned about his partner's health.

> Research suggests that women with supportive partners have fewer health problems during pregnancy and more positive feelings about their changing bodies.

Whether it is you or your partner or both who are experiencing mixed emotions, the best way to deal with these anxieties is to talk about them, either together or with a trusted friend or professional. Discussion brings enlightenment and understanding. Your partner can scarcely be expected to understand your concerns or the physical and psychological mood swings you are undergoing if you do not voice them. By the same token, your man's fears of change and responsibility will become clear to you only if he talks about them.

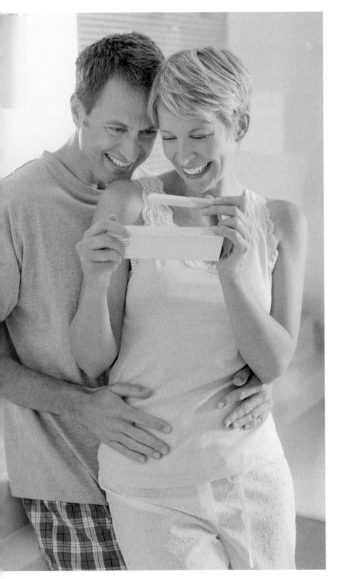

Physical Anxieties

Of course, every pregnant woman worries. It's natural. You worry about miscarriage, about the baby's development, and about the labor. But try to keep your anxieties in perspective. Drinking soothing herbal teas, such as chamomile or lime flower, can help alleviate anxiety. You can also try many of the relaxation techniques and therapies mentioned on pages 36–37.

As you get nearer to the delivery date, you will probably experience some fear about the birth. For some, this is a mild concern about the unknown, but for others it is a genuine terror of pain and how they will cope. These are not irrational fears, and people who dismiss them as such are being unhelpful. The birth is a daunting prospect, but it is also an inevitable outcome of the pregnancy and trying to be fatalistic about it can help.

Also, try talking to other mothers whom you trust to be kind and truthful about their experiences. Birth horror stories are not constructive and usually exaggerated, so politely thank the doom mongers but stop them before they get into the gory details.

Essentially, however pleased you are about the pregnancy, you or your partner should not feel at all guilty if you also experience some emotional turmoil about the coming event. Pregnancy is a time of great emotional and physical change. It is the precursor of even greater transformations in your lives once the baby arrives, and any change of this magnitude should be met with excitement and a small but healthy measure of trepidation.

greenfile

Essential oils, such as tangerine, rosemary, chamomile, and lavender, can be used in the bath or as a massage oil to alleviate anxiety and aid relaxation. The Bach Rescue Remedy is also very useful (see page 117).

Your Sex Life

It's a pretty sure bet that if you experience nausea in the first few months of your pregnancy, you are not going to feel like a rampant sex life. However, morning sickness notwithstanding, there is no reason why you should not enjoy a healthy sex life throughout your pregnancy.

Pregnancy is a nine-month continuum, and there may be times when you feel sexy and times when you don't. Rest assured, though, that it is perfectly safe to make love throughout the nine months—research does not show any increased risk of miscarriage from having sex.

Yet another common worry—especially among men—is that sex during pregnancy might hurt the baby. However, the amniotic fluid that surrounds the baby is there to protect and cushion against external bumps and bashes, so the baby cannot be harmed when you make love. In the extremely rare event that your baby is at risk due to your having a low-lying placenta, for example, your doctor or midwife should detect this and give you the relevant advice.

Although there may be times when you lose interest in sex, particularly in the first and last weeks, making love can be particularly enjoyable during pregnancy. You become aroused more easily as a result of the increase in hormone levels and the spontaneity resulting from no contraceptive concerns.

As you get larger, however, you may need to revise the positions you use in lovemaking. If the bump gets in the way of the traditional man-on-top position, try sitting astride his lap, kneeling with him behind, or lying side by side like spoons. This position is particularly effective in later pregnancy because your weight is supported.

greenfile
Many women swear that if the baby is overdue, having sex can induce labor, although there is no scientific evidence to support this claim.

Emotional Support

Even the most longed-for pregnancy brings with it concerns, stresses, and pressures for both parents. So this is a time when, as a couple, you need to reevaluate your needs and expectations regarding emotional support.

Irrespective of whether or not you are enjoying an active sex life, it is important that you discuss how you feel emotionally and sexually as openly as possible and from the heart. Each partner needs to listen to and nurture the other's emotional needs and expectations, but you must also feel free to express how you feel in response.

Sometimes, if a pregnant woman is less interested in intimacy, her partner can feel rejected. By the same token, if she perceives that her partner finds her growing and changing body unattractive, this can be extremely hurtful. These sexual tensions need to be discussed between you before they grow out of all proportion.

Of course, if your sexual needs differ at this time, there are other alternatives that can sustain intimacy and a loving relationship. Cuddling, stroking, and massage are all alternatives to sexual intercourse that can keep a committed, loving relationship on an even keel.

A final, gentle word of warning: many pregnant women fall into the trap of expecting their partner to anticipate their new needs during pregnancy, whether these are physical, emotional, and/or sexual. However, your partner cannot read your mind, so you must share your expectations and desires with him, so that he can respond—hopefully empathetically and lovingly.

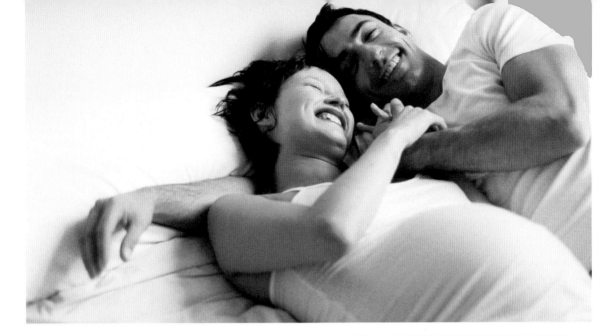

Post-baby Sex

Without wishing to get ahead of ourselves, it's worth giving a little thought in advance to resuming your sex life after the baby is born, for you can become pregnant again very soon after the birth. As to when it's safe to resume your sex life, this is entirely down to personal circumstances and preferences. You should not have sex if you are still discharging—and most women don't want to have sex at this time anyway—but otherwise, you can have sex as soon as you both feel ready. Your doctor or midwife will be happy to discuss contraception choices with you.

cervical cap check

If you used a diaphragm or cervical cap before you became pregnant, check with your doctor or planned parenthood center to make sure it still fits after the birth of your baby, since your vagina and cervix change shape during pregnancy and birth. If you later lose or gain more than 7 lb (3 kg), get the fitting checked again.

greenfile

Breast-feeding can act as a very effective contraceptive only if you are fully breast-feeding a baby under six months—i.e. you must be breast-feeding at regular intervals, day and night; giving your baby no other food or drink, so no breast-feeds are missed; and having no periods. Research shows that there is a 1–2 percent failure rate with fully breast-feeding, which is comparable to that with condoms. But you have to follow the rules. If you don't want to take any risk whatsoever, use contraception.

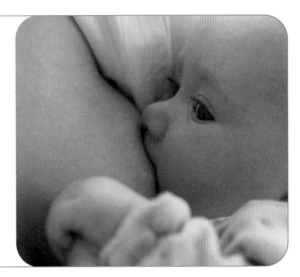

Relaxation Techniques

Pregnancy is a time of unknowns and uncertainties. Women who have been in control of their lives can be disconcerted by the feeling that the events of pregnancy are unfolding beyond their control. Add in the cocktail of hormones coursing through the body, which can cause a bewildering spectrum of emotions in quick succession, and you can see why some women find pregnancy stressful.

Yoga

Yoga is ideal for expectant women and new mothers, as it strengthens, tones, and relaxes the body and mind. It is also excellent for opening up the pelvis before the birth.

One of the most popular forms of yoga in the West is hatha yoga, which uses postures (asanas) and breathing techniques (pranayamas) to help you to become calm and relaxed. There are other forms of yoga; some more esoteric forms concentrate on the body's energy centers (chakras) and the flow of life energy (prana) through the physical and nonphysical or "subtle" bodies, often incorporating meditation and visualization into the practice.

> **WARNING** After 30 weeks, you should not attempt the yoga positions that are performed on your back.

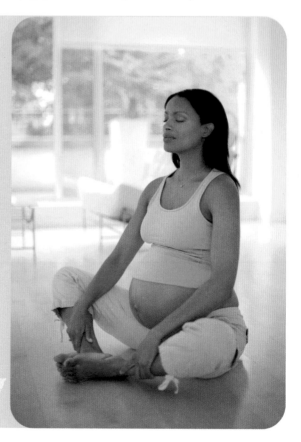

COBBLER'S OR TAILOR'S POSE (BADDHA KONASANA)

The following pose is excellent for opening the hips and pelvis in readiness for the birth.

Sit with your back straight and legs outstretched in front of you.

Bend the knees, bringing the soles of your feet together and letting your knees fall out to either side.

Keep your spine long, and press the outer edges of the feet together strongly.

Don't force the knees down or bounce them; instead let them fall until they reach a comfortable level. With practice, they will go farther.

Tip: If it helps, you can put some padding under your seat bones, and position a block under each knee for support, if necessary.

Whichever form of yoga you choose, it can be highly beneficial for aiding relaxation and alleviating various pregnancy ailments, such as backache, joint pain, depression, and respiratory problems.

It is recommended that you find a class that is specifically designed for pregnant women; or, at the very least, make sure that your teacher is aware of your situation so she can suggest positions that are comfortable and appropriate for pregnancy.

Some teachers recommend that you avoid using yoga in the first trimester of your pregnancy. You should never practise yoga if you are in pain or unwell, and stop if any position becomes uncomfortable.

Meditation and Visualization

You can deepen your state of relaxation by using meditative and relaxation techniques. There are various recognized forms of meditation, but most rely on the principle of emptying your mind of clutter and focusing on a specific thought or image, such as a flower or candle. Sometimes a word or mantra is repeated to help focus the mind.

Research shows that during meditation, the brain produces alpha brainwaves, evoking a state of deep relaxation, lowering blood pressure, and decreasing muscle tension.

There are numerous meditation CDs and DVDs available to guide you through the process, or you could consult a practitioner.

Visualization is similar to meditation, but rather than focusing on a single thought or image, you picture a positive scenario or outcome for a situation that is worrying you. For example, you might visualize a swift and straightforward birth, or you might picture

CONNECTING WITH YOUR BABY

The following visualization exercise is designed to help you connect with your unborn baby:

Sit in a comfortable, quiet place where you won't be interrupted.

Slow your breathing until it becomes rhythmic and steady: breathe in through the nose and out through the mouth.

Place your hands on either side of your "bump."

Focus on your breath, and visualize it spreading from your lungs, through your bloodstream, and into your baby, energizing him.

As you exhale, see the air leaving your body, taking stress and anxiety with it as you blow out.

Continue for as long as is comfortable. When you are ready to stop, slowly open your eyes and bring your consciousness back to the room.

As your breathing returns to normal, you can resume your normal activities.

NOTE As your energized breath reaches your baby, he may respond to it by wriggling or turning inside the womb.

your unborn child and think about the positive future you will have together. Alternatively, you may choose to imagine a calming scene, such as a palm-fringed beach or a flower-strewn mountainside, to relieve stress.

WARNING Meditation and visualization are powerful tools for relaxation. However, if you are at all concerned about the techniques involved, or if you experience any disturbing images, please consult a qualified practitioner or your doctor.

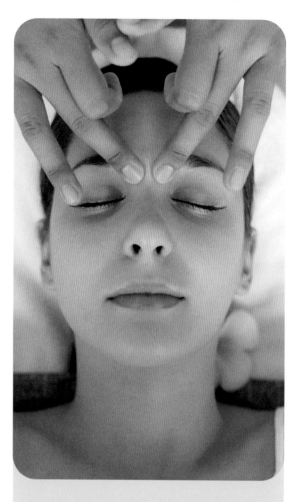

Massage

Throughout history, pregnant women have regularly been given massage by their midwives and caregivers; and in some traditional societies this practice persists today. It is believed that massaging the body, especially the tummy, hips, and legs, allows the mother to relax but also to become comfortable with and aware of her changing shape.

Massage also gives traditional midwives the opportunity to check routinely on the baby's position and, toward the latter stages of pregnancy, to massage the baby into the correct position if necessary.

In the developed world, sadly, massage is not an integral part of prenatal care, but it is still hugely beneficial. A full massage has a similar effect to doing exercise: it stimulates blood flow, which in turn oxygenates the mother's and baby's bodies. This helps to reduce fatigue, listlessness, nausea, and even mild depression.

A regular massage, provided by either your partner, a friend, or a professional massage therapist, will help you to relax deeply. It can be especially helpful to those experiencing sleep problems during pregnancy. Massage can also help to relieve general pregnancy problems, ranging from general aches and pains to backache and headache.

It doesn't matter that your partner may not be formally trained in massage. A simple back or belly rub or a foot massage each night is great for keeping intimacy alive, especially if you are not interested in sex at this time. It also gives your partner a chance to feel close to the growing baby, as well as releasing tension for you.

If you don't have anyone whom you trust to give you a massage, all is not lost. You can always enjoy the same benefits by giving yourself a massage (see right), although you cannot effectively massage the upper back this way. Nonetheless, this is a great way to relax yourself, to ease aches and pains, and to communicate with your baby.

AROMATHERAPY OILS TO AVOID DURING PREGNANCY

If massaging directly onto the skin, it is safe to use carrier oil. Seek advice if you wish to add a few drops of aromatherapy oils.

However, the following oils should be avoided during pregnancy:

aniseed, arnica, basil, clary sage, cypress, fennel, jasmine, juniper, marjoram, rosemary

WARNING Massage is usually safe for most pregnant women, although it is advisable to check with your doctor prior to having one. If you have high blood pressure or diabetes, prenatal massage is not recommended.

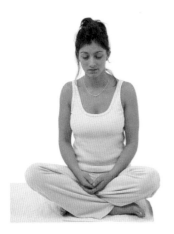

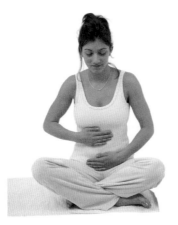

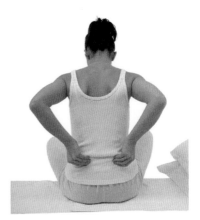

1 Begin the massage by sitting comfortably on the floor in a warm room. You can be clothed; or you may prefer to use a pure carrier oil, such as sunflower, sweet almond, or grapeseed oil, to rub directly onto your naked skin.

2 Place the palm of both hands on your stomach and, using light circular movements, gently massage the whole area. Use only as much pressure as is comfortable, and don't forget to breathe naturally.

3 After several minutes, bring your hands behind your back with your thumbs facing down toward your abdomen and fingers resting on your lower back. With the flats of your fingers, make light circular strokes all over your lower back. Stretch only as far as you can comfortably reach; this will vary as the pregnancy progresses.

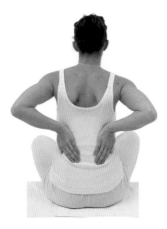

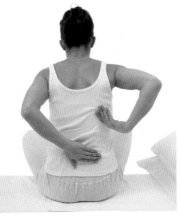

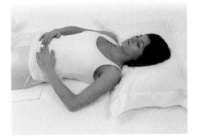

4 Using the flat or the back of your hands, rub up and down, or use the fingertips to ease areas of tension in your lower back.

5 Finally, stroke up from your buttocks to your waist in an alternate-hand stroking movement.

6 Now, lie down and rest with your hands, palms facing down, just below your navel. As your bump gets bigger, you may be more comfortable lying on your side. Don't forget to talk to your baby as you massage. You may like to play some soothing music in the background and dim the lights for complete relaxation.

A Healthy Start 39

Miscarriage

Sadly, up to one in four pregnancies in the United States ends in a miscarriage. However, most miscarriages happen before the twelfth week, and after that period they are relatively rare. Still, a miscarriage can be devastating for both parents, however early it occurs.

The cause of these miscarriages is rarely known, but rest assured it is extremely unlikely to be anything you have done or not done. Whether you stayed in bed from the day of your positive pregnancy test or spent every day mountain biking, it wouldn't change things. It's nature's way of making sure that when you do have a baby, it has the best chance for all of its life.

If a miscarriage should, unfortunately, happen to you, it is important that you and your partner be able to address your feelings of loss and, if necessary, allow yourselves a period of bereavement.

Although it may be painful to discuss, it can be extremely valuable to talk about your loss to your family doctor or another health professional, or contact the American Pregnancy Association (see Useful Contacts, page 156). Professional counseling may also be helpful and advisable in some cases. Single mothers, in particular, may well benefit from additional emotional support.

Support for Fathers

Since it is the woman who goes through the physical process of miscarriage and undergoes any medical intervention (she may need an operation or medical treatment to empty her womb), the focus of attention tends to fall on her.

Yet the father can be just as devastated—both mentally and emotionally—so try to ensure that you both seek support.

It is also common for the man to feel the need "to be strong" for you, and consequently not show how badly he is hurting, which may appear as being uncaring. So try to be honest with each other and share your feelings.

Remembering Your Baby

Although the risk of miscarriage decreases dramatically after 12 weeks of pregnancy, in rare cases it can still happen up to week 24 (after which time it is known as a stillbirth.) In the case of a late miscarriage, many parents benefit from being helped to remember their baby in some way, and over the last decade many hospitals have developed more sensitive procedures for dealing with these issues.

The following provisions are offered by some hospitals. In later miscarriages, some hospitals will take a photograph of the baby for you. Others may offer a hand- or footprint. You may be able to arrange for the hospital chaplain or a representative from your own faith to give a short service, prayer, or blessing for your baby. Some hospitals arrange regular services of remembrance or have a Garden or Book of Remembrance in which your baby's details can be entered.

There's no ruling for what happens to your baby's body if you deliver before 24 weeks (unless there are signs of life), but hospitals may offer a choice of cremation or burial. If parents want a burial or cremation, or want to take away fetal remains to dispose of themselves (in accordance with environmental regulations and the law in their state), they should discuss this with the hospital.

Recovery Time

After the miscarriage, a D&C (dilation and curettage) or evacuation is carried out to reduce the chance of infection and ensure that you don't continue bleeding over the following weeks. The D&C doesn't weaken your cervix or make you more likely to miscarry in subsequent pregnancies.

You may bleed for up to two weeks, and possibly experience cramping pains. If the pain is severe or the blood loss very heavy, contact your doctor without delay. It's advisable to use pads rather than tampons and to refrain from sex until the bleeding has stopped, to avoid the risk of infection. You should get your next period in four to six weeks after the miscarriage.

How quickly you return to normal activities depends on the individual. You can expect to feel physically low for a week or so, and you should try to take things easy during this time. Do not attempt to return to work until you feel physically and emotionally strong, unless you find the routine, the support and sympathy of colleagues, and the focus of work helpful.

Doctors' opinions vary on how long you should wait before trying for another baby, but most advise that you wait until you've had at least one period. More importantly, you must feel physically and emotionally ready to try again. If you are not ready to conceive immediately, review your choice of contraception, since you can ovulate during the first weeks following your miscarriage.

Fears for the Future

After a miscarriage it is perfectly natural to worry about whether you will ever have a healthy baby, but the prospects of a successful pregnancy are better than you think; even people who have had three miscarriages still have a 60 percent chance of having a successful pregnancy next time, although this figure varies with age. In fact, medical investigations are rarely instigated until after at least three miscarriages. When you conceive again, try to take the next pregnancy one day at a time and to share your feelings and fears with your partner, friends, or doctor if it helps.

Homeopathy can be used to great effect in regard to miscarriage, not only to help with physical symptoms but also to alleviate grief (see page 114).

POSSIBLE CAUSES OF MISCARRIAGE

AGE There is a rise in miscarriage risk as maternal age increases. Women under the age of 35 have about a 15 percent chance of miscarriage. For those between 35 and 45, the risk is 20–35 percent; for those over 45 it is up to 50 percent.

GENETIC ABNORMALITY About half of all early miscarriages occur because of chance chromosome abnormalities.

WEIGHT It is important to fall within the recommended weight band for your height. Being either under- or overweight can increase the risk.

ENVIRONMENTAL HAZARDS There is a 30–50 per cent increased risk of miscarriage in women who smoke. Also, both smoking and drinking can adversely affect the quality of a man's sperm. This in turn can lead to a genetic abnormality if such sperm fertilize an egg, and so the pregnancy miscarries.

INFECTIONS A high temperature and some specific illnesses or infections, such as German measles (rubella), may cause miscarriage.

ANATOMICAL PROBLEMS If the cervix (neck of the womb) is weak, it may start to open as the uterus becomes heavier in later pregnancy, and this can lead to miscarriage.

TESTS Chorionic villus sampling (CVS) and amniocentesis, which are tests offered during some pregnancies, carry a 1–3 in 200 chance of miscarriage (see page 97).

RADIATION The jury is still out on whether or not radiation from VDUs can cause miscarriage, but enough concerns have been raised for you at least to limit the time you spend at the screen or to use a screen protector, if possible (see page 68).

greenfile

Some pregnant women are afraid that if they should have a fall or overexert themselves physically, they may miscarry, but these are not generally causes for concern. The baby is well cushioned inside the womb and should be perfectly safe. However, if you do a lot of high-impact activities, such as horse riding, running, or aerobics, you may like to consider a lower impact alternative until after the birth.

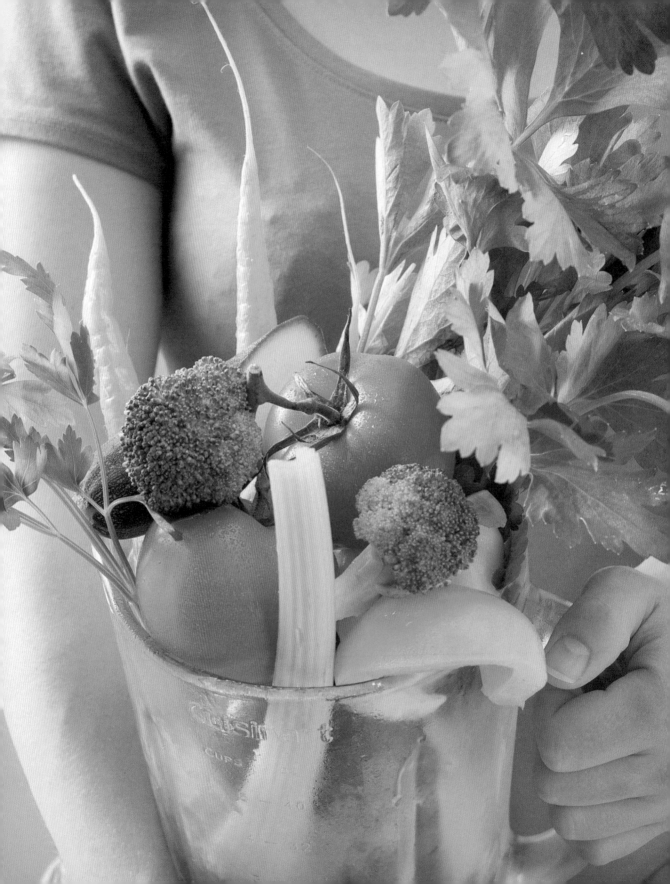

3 Healthy Eating

Eating healthily and getting the best nutrition for you and your unborn baby is important, no matter at what stage of pregnancy you are. Yet there is so much conflicting advice and so many old wives' tales about what constitutes good nutrition during pregnancy that it's easy to become confused and anxious about what you should or should not be eating.

Undoubtedly, a good balanced diet throughout your pregnancy will ensure that your baby develops as naturally and healthily as possible; and, ideally, you should start looking at your diet before you try to conceive so that you are in prime condition for the pregnancy and birth. But if the pregnancy is unplanned, it's still not too late to start with proper nutrition.

In this chapter, we look at the pregnancy superfoods (see page 44) that will give your unborn baby the best boost for optimum growth and development and at those foods and substances that you should really try to avoid (see page 50), at least for the nine months of your pregnancy.

If you follow a special diet, we will explore how best you can make that diet work for you and your baby (see page 54). We'll also look at how to deal with the thorny issues of cravings (see page 60) and weight gain in the most natural way possible.

The old adage "you are what you eat" is definitely true and never more apt than during pregnancy. So to maximize your baby's opportunity to develop healthily in the womb and to avoid disease later in life, a natural and healthy diet—plus a little treat now and then—is the way forward.

Pregnancy Superfoods

Although the overriding principle of good nutrition during pregnancy is to enjoy your food and to be realistic about what you can change in your diet in order to eat more healthily, there are certain key elements of your diet that are essential if you are to nurture a healthy pregnancy for you and your baby.

Many health professionals, including midwives, place the greatest emphasis on a handful of "superfoods," and the consensus is that while you do not need a special diet when pregnant, you should definitely include the following high-nutrient powerfoods in your daily meal planning.

Spinach

Together with broccoli and other dark green leafy vegetables, spinach is the heavyweight of superfoods for pregnant women. That's because it is rich in folic acid, also known as folate or folacin, which is one of the B group of vitamins, which is essential for your developing baby's health (see page 23).

While it is recommended that before you conceive and during the first three months of pregnancy, you take a daily folic acid supplement (see page 58), you should also make sure you include lots of folate-rich foods in your diet, too (see list, above right). Folic acid in foods is easily destroyed by overcooking, so wherever possible, either lightly steam folate-rich vegetables or eat them raw.

Other good food sources of folates:

Leafy green vegetables, including lettuce
Brussels sprouts
Baked potato
Asparagus
Broccoli
Black-eyed peas
Bran flakes
Wheatgerm
Canned salmon
Hard-boiled egg
Papaya
Orange

Watercress

Packed full of iron, this is a true pregnancy superfood. During your pregnancy, your body makes so much extra blood that your iron requirements are much greater than at any other stage in life. Iron helps red blood cells transport oxygen to all parts of the body. However, your growing fetus is also building up its own iron reserves by taking the iron from your body. If your stores of body iron become depleted, you may feel tired and lacking in energy, and you may become anemic, so make sure you get plenty of iron-rich foods in your diet.

greenfile

Thanks to Popeye, spinach is probably the best-known source of iron from our diet. Paradoxically, though, spinach contains a substance that makes it hard for the body to absorb its iron, so you're better choosing other sources if it's iron that you're after.

VITAMIN C PLUS IRON

To help your body absorb more of the iron from your diet, try combining food or drinks rich in vitamin C, such as oranges, orange juice, strawberries, kiwi fruit, bell peppers, and tomatoes, with foods rich in iron from non-meat sources.

WARNING Although liver is a good source of iron, if you're pregnant you should avoid eating it because of the amount of vitamin A it contains (see page 51).

Other good food sources of iron:

Meat, especially red meat

Beans and legumes

Nuts, such as cashews, coconut, almonds, hazelnuts, pine nuts, macadamias, and pistachios

Dried fruit, especially dried apricots

Wholegrains, such as brown rice, wholewheat pasta, and bread

Fortified breakfast cereals

Soybean flour

Most dark green leafy vegetables (such as watercress and curly kale)

Brazil Nuts

A handful of Brazil nuts each day will provide you with a good supply of zinc and selenium. During pregnancy, your body needs zinc to produce and repair DNA, the body's genetic map and basic building blocks of cells, at a time when rapid cell growth is occurring.

Other good food sources of zinc:

Fortified breakfast cereals

Baked beans

Red meat and poultry

Nuts

Wholegrains

Dairy products

Yogurt

Eating yogurt is a great way to give your calcium stores a boost, particularly if you're not fond of milk. Calcium has a number of important functions for pregnant women. Its superfood credentials include helping to build strong bones and teeth, regulating muscle

Although oysters are the richest food source of zinc, experts caution against eating raw oysters during pregnancy because of the risk of food-borne illness.

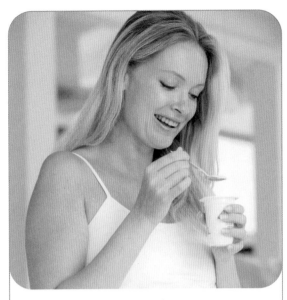

greenfile

You need vitamin D, a fat-soluble vitamin, to aid absorption of calcium in the body during pregnancy. Vitamin D is found in milk and oily fish, so try to include these in your diet alongside foods rich in calcium.

contraction, including the heartbeat, and making sure blood clots normally.

Other good food sources of calcium:

Milk

Cheese and other dairy foods

Green leafy vegetables (such as broccoli, cabbage, and okra, but not spinach)

Soy beans

Tofu

Soy drinks with added calcium

Nuts, especially almonds and Brazil nuts

Sesame seeds

Bread and anything made with fortified flour

Fish of which you eat the bones, such as sardines and canned salmon

Blueberries

A fantastic superfood at any time but especially when pregnant, blueberries are bursting with antioxidants, folates, fiber, and oodles of vitamin C, which is essential for your iron absorption and hormone production.

Other good food sources of vitamin C:

Most fruits, especially citrus and kiwi fruit
Berries, including strawberries, blackberries,
 and cherries
Potatoes
Parsley

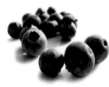

Avocados

Sliced in salads or spooned straight from the skin, this versatile fruit (yes, it is!) is packed full of vitamin E, which promotes new cell development in your baby and may help pregnant women deal with toxins.

Mothers pass vitamin E to their babies in the last 12 weeks of pregnancy (about 20 mg in total), so that is the time to stock up on avocados and other food sources of this important vitamin.

Other good food sources of vitamin E:

Plant oils, such as soy, corn, and olive oil, provide the
 richest sources

Nuts	Brussels sprouts
Soy beans	Spinach
Vegetable oil	Whole grain products
Broccoli	Eggs

> Some very premature babies (born at less than 28 weeks) can show signs of vitamin E deficiency soon after birth if they are born before the transfer from mother to baby takes place.

Sardines

If you believe the hype, foods rich in essential fatty acids (omega-3 and omega-6) are the superfoods to top all superfoods, and that's certainly true where pregnancy is concerned. Recent research suggests that pregnant women have increased need of essential fatty acids, because they are important for your baby's neurological growth and brain development.

Other good sources of essential fatty acids:

Plant oils, such as flaxseed, rapeseed, hempseed,
 soybean, cottonseed, and blackcurrant seed oil

Tuna	Nuts
Salmon	Seeds
Mackerel	
Herring	

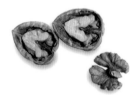

Apricots

These are the perfect pregnancy snack food. Packed full of folate, calcium, magnesium, and fiber, they are also a great source of beta-carotene, the plant-based form of vitamin A. Beta-carotene helps to strengthen your immune system and that of your developing baby. It's also beneficial for the development of your baby's skin and eyes.

> Choose naturally coloured dried apricots (preferably organic) that have not been treated with sulphur.

Other good food sources of beta-carotene:

Carrots	Collard greens
Sweet potatoes	Winter squash
Kale	Coriander
Spinach	Thyme

WARNING Extremely high doses of vitamin E have been linked with risks of internal bleeding, but since it is a fat-soluble vitamin, it is quite hard to overdose.

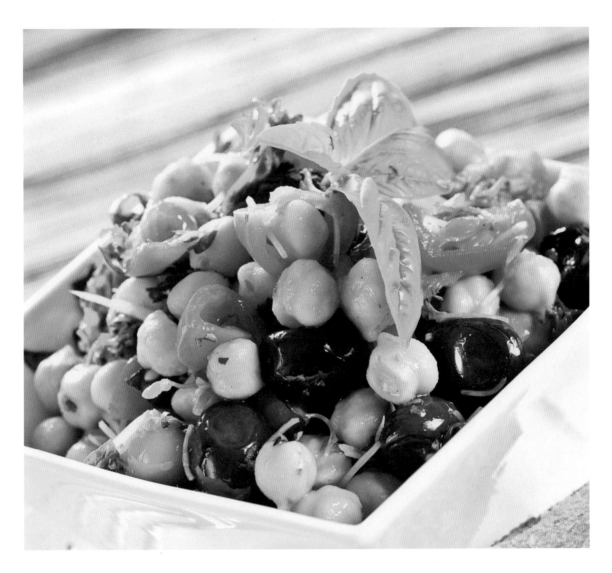

Baked Beans

It may sound like a joke, but the humble baked bean (so long as it's low-sugar) is a great source of vegetable protein, fiber, folate, and calcium. In fact, all legumes (beans, lentils, and peas) supply the amino acids that the body needs and, as such, are a cheap and nutritious pregnancy superfood that can easily be added to soups, casseroles, and curries.

greenfile

Beta-carotene is easily destroyed on cooking, so vegetables containing vitamin A should be lightly steamed or eaten raw to get the optimum nutritional value.

Other good food sources of fiber and vegetable protein:

Chickpeas	Peas
Lentils	Beans

WARNING Retinol, the animal form of vitamin A, can be harmful to unborn babies in large doses, so avoid sources such as cod-liver oil. Prenatal supplements contain the plant-derived form of vitamin A (beta-carotene), which is perfectly safe.

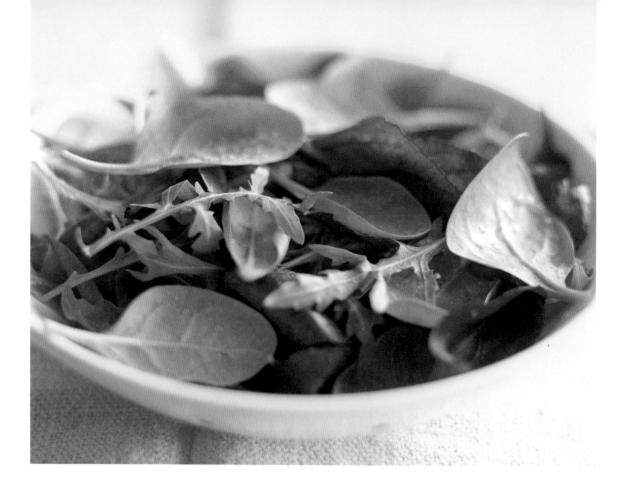

Magnesium

Often overlooked as a nutrient, magnesium is in fact classed as a pregnancy superfood because it helps to build and repair your body tissue, and a severe deficiency during pregnancy may lead to preeclampsia (high blood pressure and swelling), birth defects, and infant mortality.

While calcium stimulates muscles to contract (see Yogurt, page 45), magnesium stimulates them to relax. In this way, these two "super" minerals work in tandem. Research suggests that proper levels of magnesium during pregnancy can help keep the uterus from contracting until week 35. Conversely, a magnesium deficiency at this point could lead to premature labor.

You'll get a good natural source of magnesium from green leafy vegetables, wholegrains and wheatgerm, nuts and seeds (such as almonds and pumpkin and sunflower seeds), starches (such as pasta), and milk.

Organic Food

Although there is as yet no conclusive scientific evidence that organic food produce is either any safer or of greater nutritional value than nonorganic produce, many holistic practitioners and nutritionists still believe that organic food represents the safest option for pregnant women.

Some experts maintain that the levels of chemicals found in conventionally produced foods are perfectly safe, but even low levels of chemicals have been found to be detrimental to the health of a developing fetus and of young children, due to their sensitive, developing immune systems.

Although it is not essential to eat organically grown foods during your pregnancy (but good if you can), wherever possible or practical, you should try to choose food items that have been minimally processed, if at all, and with few or no additives or preservatives.

Top ten pregnancy superfoods

These foods are packed with vitamins, minerals, and nutrients. If you can eat some of these each day, you'll be doing yourself and your unborn baby a great service.

Bananas, oranges, and other fresh fruit

Dried apricots and prunes

Broccoli and other green vegetables

Salmon and other oily fish

Wholewheat bread and brown rice

Lean red meat, chicken, and turkey

Yogurt

Legumes, such as lentils

Fortified breakfast cereals

Nuts and seeds

Harmful Foods

The general rule of thumb during pregnancy is to eat as you would normally but to try to make sure that you have a balanced diet. For most of us, that means making an effort to eat more fruit and vegetables (five a day for optimum nutrition, and preferably organic), plenty of bread, cereals, and potatoes, together with milk and dairy foods, meat, and fish.

However, there are certain foods in a balanced diet that could be detrimental to the health of your unborn child, and these should be avoided. The vast majority of "harmful" foods fall into the category of foods that could cause an infection.

Don't be unduly alarmed, because food infections are in fact rare. However, it is only sensible to take the precaution of avoiding the foods listed here, because the effects of food infections (see page 53) can be serious for pregnant women.

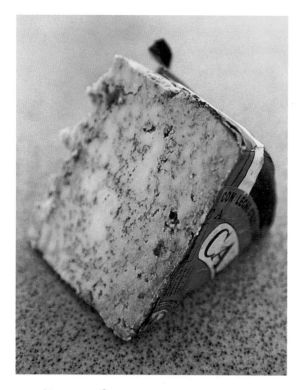

Foods to Avoid

Cheese You should avoid eating all types of mold-ripened, soft and blue-veined cheese, such as Brie, Camembert, Stilton, or Danish Blue, because of the risk of listeria (see page 53). This is a rare disease that can lead to miscarriage, stillbirth, or severe illness in your newborn baby.

Eggs If you eat eggs, make sure they are thoroughly cooked through. Avoid "runny" eggs or foods containing raw or under-cooked eggs, such as homemade mayonnaise, and certain desserts, such as tiramisu, to prevent the risk of salmonella food poisoning (see page 53).

Meat and poultry Eat only meat and poultry that is thoroughly cooked through without any traces of pink flesh or blood, and wash all surfaces and utensils after preparing raw meat. This will help to avoid infection from toxoplasma (see page 53).

Unpasteurized dairy products This does not apply to the majority of people, but just in case, make sure you do not drink unpasteurized cow's, goat's, or sheep's milk or consume their milk products.

Liver Avoid liver or liver products, such as sausages or paté, as liver can contain high levels of vitamin A, too much of which is harmful to your baby (see right).

Raw shellfish Avoid raw shellfish when you're pregnant because it can sometimes contain harmful bacteria and viruses that could cause food poisoning.

Unwashed produce Try to include more fruit, vegetables, and salads in your diet but wash them well, removing all traces of soil. This could contain toxoplasma, which can put your unborn child at risk.

Unhealthful Choices

Wherever possible, try to cut down on the amount of foods you consume containing fat, salt, or sugar. The main culprits are snack foods, such as potato chips, processed foods, such as pastries, and fast foods, such as take-out and prepackaged meals.

Salt Although salt is not restricted during pregnancy, most of us already consume more sodium than we need, so it's worth curtailing your intake. If you have a family history of high blood pressure, you may be at risk of toxemia (hypertension combined with fluid retention and protein in the urine) while you're pregnant, so discuss safe and healthy sodium levels with your doctor as early in your pregnancy as possible.

Sugar This is not unhealthful when consumed in moderation, but it does provide calories without providing any nutrients. If you are concerned about excessive weight gain during pregnancy, you should be careful not to overindulge your sweet tooth. However, you should avoid low-calorie sugar alternatives, containing artificial sweeteners, such as aspartame and saccharine, because their effects on pregnant and lactating women have not been fully studied, and there are some concerns surrounding possible health risks.

Caffeine You should also try to drink less tea, coffee, and colas, as these contain caffeine. The research regarding caffeine so far is somewhat contradictory, but one American study by the Kaiser Permanente Division of Research in 2008 has linked high caffeine consumption to an increased risk of miscarriage. The National Institutes of Health (NIH) recommends a maximum daily caffeine consumption of 300 mg during pregnancy. If you must drink coffee, try to limit yourself to a maximum of two cups per day. Better yet, you could try decaffeinated coffee and caffeine-free teas and soft drinks, or drink fruit or herbal teas.

VITAMIN A

A normal supply of vitamin A is critical for embryonic development and is a requirement for brain development, particularly in its early stages.

It's actually quite easy to get vitamin A from your diet, since it's widely available in meat, dairy, fish, eggs, and fortified cereals in the form of "preformed vitamin A," as well as in most fruits and vegetables in the form of beta-carotene (a nutrient that is converted to vitamin A by your body as needed).

The trick during pregnancy is not to consume too much of the preformed vitamin A, which in high doses can cause birth defects and liver toxicity, with an increased risk of miscarriage. The U.S. government considers 3,000 mcg RAE (10,000 IU) the maximum amount of preformed vitamin A you should take in from supplements, animal sources, and fortified foods each day, but you can still get as much beta-carotene as you want from fruits and vegetables.

So be careful if you take any supplements that your practitioner doesn't recommend, as some over-the-counter brands of multivitamins contain excessive amounts of preformed vitamin A.

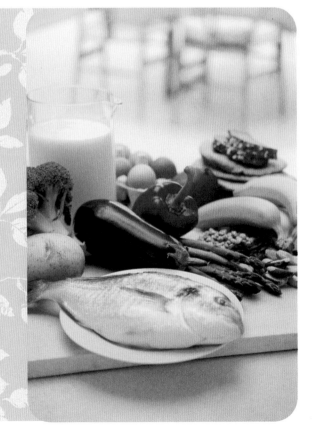

Alcohol

Advice from the Centers of Disease Control and Prevention (see Useful Contacts, page 156) is that you should not drink alcohol at all if you are pregnant or trying to become pregnant. It is known that if you drink heavily you have an increased risk of miscarriage, and alcohol can cause serious harm to the baby's growth and brain development. A British study has shown that:

- Pregnant women who drink more than 63 oz (1,875 ml) of wine or 13 oz (375 ml) of spirits a week have an increased risk of having a baby with a low birth weight.
- Pregnant women who drink more than 84 oz (2,500 ml) of wine or 17 oz (500 ml) of spirits a week have an increased risk of having a baby with some damage to the brain, causing impaired intellect.
- Pregnant women who drink very heavily risk having a baby with fetal alcohol syndrome. Babies with this syndrome have brain damage, a low birth weight, and facial malformations.

Since the exact amount of alcohol that is safe during pregnancy is unknown, the safest option is not to drink at all. Your baby is most vulnerable to alcohol during the very early stages of pregnancy, so it is just as important to avoid alcohol when you are trying to become pregnant. If you are going to have an occasional drink during your pregnancy, doing so after the twelfth week is considered to be less of a risk. If you do choose to drink alcohol when you are pregnant, limit your consumption to one or perhaps two drinks a week—that is a very small glass of wine, or about 10 oz (300 ml) of beer, or a small measure of spirits. And never get drunk.

If you find it difficult to stop drinking alcohol, seek advice and help from your doctor or midwife.

Women metabolize alcohol more slowly than men do because they tend to have smaller livers and more body fat.

Peanuts

In the past, some nutritionists recommended that you avoid peanuts and food containing peanut products, such as peanut butter and unrefined peanut oil, during pregnancy if you or the baby's father has a history of asthma, hay fever, eczema, or other allergies, in order to reduce the risk of your baby's developing a peanut allergy in later life. Scientific evidence varies with regard to this matter, but in 2009 a British government investigation concluded that it is safe to eat peanuts and peanut products during pregnancy (see page 56).

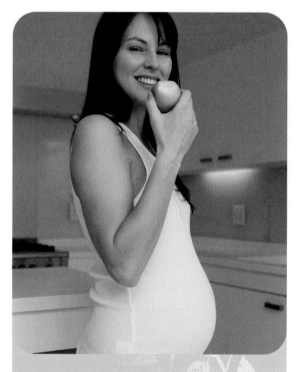

"EATING FOR TWO"
The sad news for foodies is that you can forget the old adage of "eating for two." You don't have to increase your food intake during pregnancy—your energy requirements are about 1,940 calories per day, increasing by only 200 calories in the third trimester.

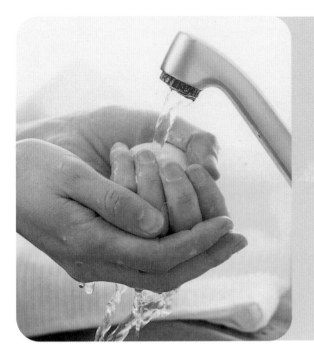

GOOD FOOD HYGIENE

Do not allow frozen food to defrost in transit before putting into the freezer; observe use-by dates.

Chilled food must be thoroughly rewarmed to prevent salmonella infection.

Regular hand-washing is essential, especially after using the toilet, handling animals or soil, and before preparing or eating food; wash hands after handling raw foods.

Keep raw and cooked food separate; also utensils, such as chopping boards.

Do not reheat food more than once.

Food Infections

Salmonella This is the most common cause of food poisoning, but it does not cross the placenta, so although you may be very unwell, your baby should not be harmed by a salmonella food infection. In exceptionally rare cases, there have been reports of neonatal infection, miscarriage, and premature labor.

Toxoplasmosis This is a more serious infection if you are pregnant. It is caused by a parasite picked up by handling or eating raw or under-cooked meat or touching infected cat feces. The infection can cross the placenta and cause miscarriage or deformities. Your baby is at the greatest risk at 10–24 weeks. Treatment for toxoplasmosis during pregnancy is also problematical because the drugs used can adversely affect the fetus.

Listeriosis Perhaps the most serious food infection of them all, listeriosis, resulting from eating soft cheese or under-cooked chicken, is thankfully rare (1 in 10,000 pregnancies). If you are infected, the bacterium can cross the placenta, causing spontaneous abortion in the first trimester of pregnancy or premature labor in the second trimester. The bacteria can survive in temperatures as low as 39°F (4°C), so make sure your fridge is turned down below this level.

greenfile

If you do suffer from a mild gastrointestinal upset from something you've eaten, try sipping a herbal infusion or tea. Aniseed, fennel, mint, ginger, or chamomile are all very calming for an upset stomach. See page 120 for homemade ginger tea.

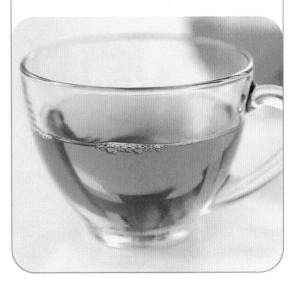

Special Dietary Needs

If you follow a special diet, either as a lifestyle choice or for health reasons, you may be concerned about getting the necessary nutrients for your growing baby. In fact, so long as you pay attention to what you are eating and plan ahead, it is possible to meet all your nutritional needs (and those of your unborn child) while eating many special diets, including vegan, diabetic, and macrobiotic.

Indeed, some people believe that a vegetarian diet is healthier during pregnancy, as the foods you eat are less likely to be overprocessed or to include so much fat, additives, or chemicals.

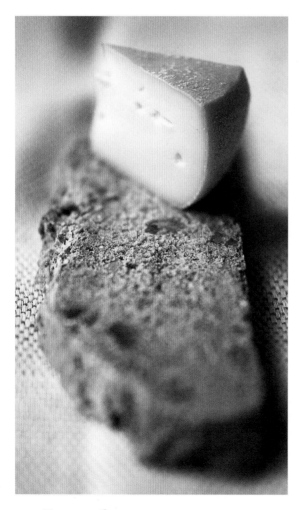

Nonetheless, you should be aware of certain nutritional pitfalls associated with these diets during pregnancy so that you can make provisions to compensate.

Vegetarian

The primary concern for you as a pregnant vegetarian woman is that you get enough protein and, if you don't eat dairy, calcium too.

Protein can be found in cereals, legumes (beans), nuts, seeds, eggs, soy, and Quorn, but protein is not well stored in the body, and you need a good supply of it. To improve your ability to get adequate protein from a vegetarian diet, you should combine sources for optimum effect. So, grains can be combined with smaller amounts of beans or legumes (or dairy products if this applies); and nuts and seeds can be combined with beans or legumes.

greenfile

Ultimately, whichever diet you follow, remember to listen to your body at this time. If you suddenly feel a desire to change or supplement your usual diet during your pregnancy, you should go with the flow. And try to resist the temptation to beat yourself up about breaking your normal dietary rules—after all, these are choices and not written in stone, and you can always revert to your normal code of eating once the baby is born, if you so desire.

Still short of ideas? Well, why not try rice and beans, rice and tahini, or macaroni and cheese for dinner? Peanut butter on wholewheat toast or a cookie containing peanuts and sunflower seeds make a protein-packed snack.

Similarly, vegetarians who eat little dairy produce and vegans need to be particularly careful to get enough calcium in the diet. A good intake of calcium-rich foods, such as green leafy vegetables, almonds, sesame seeds or tahini, cow's milk, fortified soy milk, tofu, hard cheese, bread, and yogurt, can be

greenfile
Iron absorption is increased if iron-rich foods are eaten with a good source of vitamin C (found in fresh fruit and vegetables). See also page 44.

improved still further by combining them with vitamin D, which aids calcium absorption. Vitamin D can be obtained from sunlight, margarine, dairy products, and some fortified breakfast cereals.

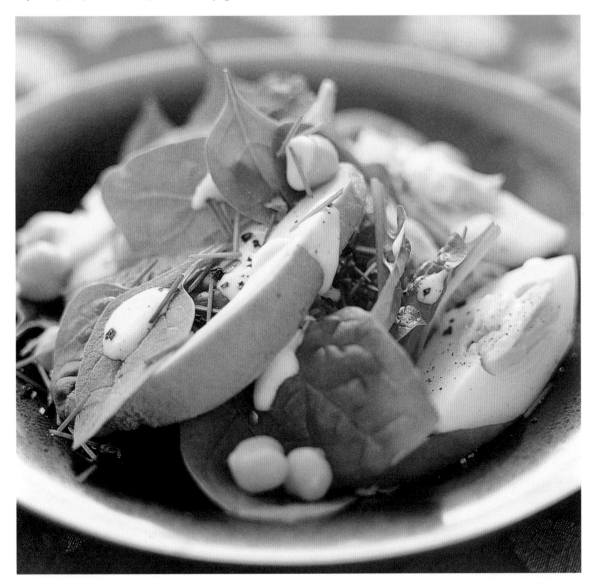

Finally, iron levels normally decrease during pregnancy, but vegetarian women are particularly susceptible. Make sure you are getting plenty of iron-rich vegetarian foods, such as whole-grain cereals, legumes, leafy green vegetables, nuts, dried fruits, and fortified breakfast cereals.

Don't forget, too, that if you are a vegetarian who relies mainly on prepackaged foods, these have still been processed, and some of the nutrients of freshly prepared meals will be missing.

If you have any concerns about whether your vegetarian, vegan, macrobiotic, or raw-food diet is not providing you with sufficient nutrients, you should speak to your obstetrician, or consult a dietician or nutritionist.

SPECIALIZED DIETS

If you follow any specialized diet while pregnant, it is important that you eat a wide variety of foods to get optimum nutrition, and that you follow the same health advice given to the general population.

VARIATIONS ON VEGETARIAN DIETS

Vegetarian—eats no meat or fish

Lacto-ovo vegetarian—eats no meat but eats dairy products and eggs

Lacto vegetarian—eats dairy but no meat or eggs

Vegan—eats no animal products whatsoever (sometimes including honey)

Macrobiotic—eats whole grains, beans, vegetables, sea vegetables, seeds, and nuts, and occasionally fruits in season

Raw food—eats only nonanimal foods in a raw state, in particular, fruits, vegetables, fresh juices, sprouts, nuts, and seeds

---

Diabetic Diet

When you become pregnant, the hormones released by the placenta create a resistance to insulin. As a result, it's estimated that between 2–4 percent of women develop temporary diabetes, known as gestational diabetes. This is normally detected by blood-sugar-level checks taken between 24 and 28 weeks.

If you have diabetes before pregnancy or develop gestational diabetes, you will receive dietary advice from your health professionals. This will probably include eating regular meals that are lower in fat, reducing the amount of salt in your diet and eating plenty of fruit and vegetables. You will also be encouraged to participate in low-impact activities, such as walking, swimming, yoga, or pilates.

Food Intolerance and Allergies

Although some scientific opinion recommends that women avoid eating allergenic foods, such as cow's milk, hen's eggs, and nuts, while pregnant or breast-feeding, to avoid the risk of the baby's developing an allergy to them, recent studies have discounted this risk. For example, the British Department of Health (see page 52) has concluded that peanuts are safe to eat, even by women who have a family history of allergies.

However, other precautions may need to be observed in the case of women with severely allergic parents or siblings. It's still recommended that pregnant women avoid cigarette smoking and prepare to breast-feed exclusively for at least 4–6 months.

Nonetheless, it has to be said that many women prefer to err on the safe side. If you prefer to avoid certain known allergens during pregnancy, this cannot harm your unborn child, so long as you are eating an otherwise well-balanced, nutritionally sound diet.

---

greenfile

Since diabetic women have higher levels of blood glucose, which the baby stores as body fat, statistically, they are more likely to give birth to a bigger baby.

GESTATIONAL DIABETES

There is an increased risk of diabetes during pregnancy if:

You are overweight.

You smoke or are around smokers more than average.

You are over 30.

You have a family history of diabetes.

You are from certain ethnic minorities.

You have a previous history of giving birth to a large baby (more than 10 lb [4.5 kg].)

Reducing Sugar Intake

If you have diabetes or gestational diabetes, or if sugar is detected in your urine, try to cut down on certain foods.

Foods to Avoid:

Sugary foods, such as cookies, cake, and other desserts, and some canned foods

Carbonated and sweetened soft drinks

Fatty or highly processed foods

Salt and salty foods

Foods to Eat Freely:

Carbohydrates (bread, pasta, rice, noodles, and cereals)

Fruit, vegetables, and legumes

Low-fat foods

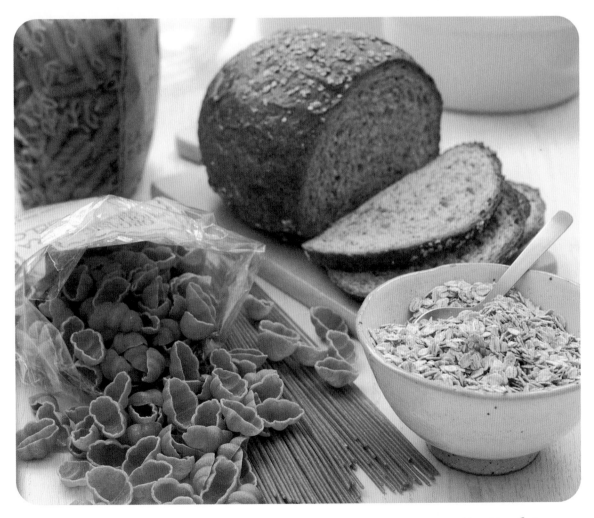

Supplements

Medical opinion on the value of vitamin supplements during pregnancy has shifted over the years. The American College of Obstetricians and Gynecologists (ACOG) has long taken the view that if you were a healthy, low-risk-pregnancy woman eating a balanced diet, routine multivitamin supplementation was not necessary. Today, it gives cautious approval to multivitamins that contain iron and folic acid.

In Britain, the Royal College of Obstetricians and Gynaecologists now encourages pregnant women to take a multivitamin supplement, recommending one brand specially formulated for pregnancy. Discuss the matter with your own doctor to make sure you get the right extra nutrients.

Folic Acid Supplements

The one piece of supplement advice that is agreed upon on both sides of the Atlantic is that when you're pregnant (or if you're trying to conceive), you should take a daily 400 mcg folic acid supplement until the twelfth week of your pregnancy. Folic acid has been shown to reduce the risk of neural tube defects, such as spina bifida. Women are advised to start taking these supplements from the time they stop using contraception, because folic acid is particularly important in early pregnancy; but it is never too late to start.

The safety of folic acid was evaluated by Britain's independent Expert Group on Vitamins and Minerals (EVM). The EVM concluded that taking folic acid supplements of up to 1 mg (1,000 mcg) per day is unlikely to do you any harm. Women who are at high risk of having a baby affected by a neural tube defect might be advised by their doctor to take more than 1 mg per day of folic acid. If this affects you, seek advice from your doctor.

Omega-3

You may have heard that the omega-3 fatty acids contained in fish oil supplements can improve a baby's cognitive development (ability to learn). This may well be the case, but there is currently not enough medical evidence to support this claim, and more research needs to be carried out to verify this theory. Until then, fish-liver oil supplements should be avoided during pregnancy because they contain high levels of vitamin A, which can be harmful to a developing baby (see page 51).

This is not to say that you should not eat fish while you are pregnant. Fish is an excellent source of protein, vitamins, and minerals, including omega-3. The British Food Standards Agency (FSA) advises that pregnant women who eat a balanced diet do not need to take fish oil supplements because eating a range of fresh fish offers more nutrients than taking supplements alone.

There are non-fish sources of omega-3 fatty acids, such as flax and hemp seeds, but the primary type of

> It is almost impossible for pregnant women to get the full, recommended amount of folic acid from food, which is why the government advises pregnant women to take folic acid supplements.

WARNING If you have diabetes, epilepsy, or celiac disease, you may need to have a higher dose of folic acid. Your doctor or midwife will be able to advise you.

omega-3 fat in these sources is alpha-linolenic acid (ALA). While the body can convert ALA into the more bioactive omega-3 fatty acids called EPA and DHA, the conversion is very inefficient. We get much more benefit from fish oil, which already contain EPA and DHA.

If you still wish to maximize the effects of omega-3 on your baby's brain development, what you're really after is a non-fish source for EPA and DHA. Certain algae, such as spirulina (see below), are high in both EPA and DHA and offer your best option for non-fish-sourced omega-3.

Vitamin D

Some obstetricians recommend that women at risk of vitamin D deficiency during pregnancy should take a 10 mcg supplement of vitamin D per day. The at-risk group may include women of South Asian, African, Caribbean, or Middle Eastern family origin, those who have limited exposure to sunlight, women who eat a diet that is particularly low in vitamin D and women with pre-pregnancy obesity. If you fall into any of those categories, you should seek advice from your prenatal care team about vitamin D supplementation.

Natural Supplementation

If your diet is healthy and balanced, you may prefer to boost your nutrition by consuming concentrated food sources. For example, spirulina, a blue-green algae, is a useful source of extra protein, especially for vegetarians, and can be taken in powder or tablet form. Molasses is an excellent source of calcium, iron, and B vitamins. You can have a tablespoon a day, eaten straight from the jar, or taken in hot water or added to a smoothie. Similarly, liquid chlorophyll is a rich source of iron (take one tablespoon a day).

greenfile

Some women claim that taking vitamin B6 reduces the severity of the nauseous feelings you get from morning sickness, although it doesn't seem to relieve the vomiting.

BANANA AND MOLASSES SMOOTHIE

This delicious smoothie gives you a boost of super-nutritious molasses, and it tastes like cappuccino!

5 pitted prunes
1 medium banana, peeled and cut into 1-in (2.5-cm) pieces
2 cups low-fat vanilla soy milk
1 tablespoon blackstrap molasses
¼ teaspoon ground cardamom
3 ice cubes

Place prunes in small bowl and cover with hot tap water. Leave for 15 minutes until plump. Drain. Combine plumped prunes and remaining ingredients in blender and blitz until smooth. If you're feeling decadent, add a scoop of vanilla ice cream.

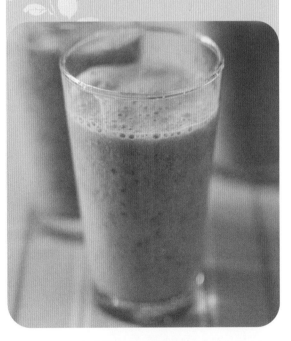

If you decide to take supplements, choose a specially formulated prenatal or pregnancy multivitamin to ensure that you do not exceed any of the recommended daily allowances during pregnancy.

Cravings

We've all heard stories of pregnant women who suddenly start to crave certain foodstuffs in the middle of the night, or who can't get enough of some unusual food combinations, such as ice cream and pickled onions. In fact, you've probably heard tell of women who even want to eat peculiar nonfood items, such as wallpaper, coal, or chalk. Although these fancies during pregnancy undoubtedly happen, the wackier cravings are actually very rare.

In general, food cravings tend to be either for sweet foods or for a favorite childhood dish. In my case, while pregnant with my second child, I had an overwhelming desire to eat milky juice bars, but thankfully, it lasted only a few days.

No one actually knows for certain what causes food cravings. Many nutritionists suspect that cravings are in response to a temporary deficiency in certain nutrients. Certainly, it is worth using a craving as a timely reminder to take a closer look at what you eat. You may find that due to morning sickness, for example, you're skipping meals and snacking instead, and this means you're missing out on a balanced diet. If your diet is deficient in some way, try to redress the balance, or ask your doctor or pharmacist to recommend a suitable vitamin or mineral supplement to take during pregnancy.

If you are craving chocolate each afternoon, it may simply mean that your body needs more energy. Perhaps carrying a snack with you, such as a sandwich, a cereal bar, or some fruit, will satisfy your body's craving for energy. If you're still hungry or craving chocolate a short while after eating a more healthful snack, then by all means, have a little of what you crave.

Other experts believe that cravings are a result of an emotional response to pregnancy—either conscious or subconscious. You may crave a childhood food that is comforting, or perhaps a food that reminds you of your cultural or religious background, especially if you

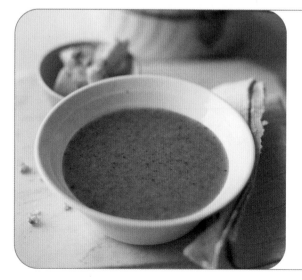

greenfile

Women suffering from iron deficiency during pregnancy sometimes develop cravings for nonfood items, such as clay, dirt, cornstarch, and ice. If you suddenly find yourself wanting to eat one of these odd items, have a blood test to check for iron-deficiency anemia. If you have a low hemoglobin count, you may be prescribed daily iron supplements, but you should certainly eat iron-rich foods.

are removed from your family. Cravings can also be ascribed to an unconscious need to honor privately your new special state of pregnancy.

Common Dislikes

In reality, rather than craving particular foods, many women actually find they go off certain foods or drinks, or other tastes. Common dislikes include toothpaste; coffee, tea, and alcohol; rich, creamy foods; and fried foods. Often, the very smell of these items is enough to make susceptible pregnant women feel quite nauseous, so it's small wonder that this symptom is often related to pregnancy sickness, which some believe is the body's way of making you eat more wisely.

Whether you crave foods or find that you suddenly dislike certain foods, this may be as a result of the fact that your senses of taste and smell are changed in pregnancy. Some women report that these senses are dulled, while others report an odd metallic taste in their mouths in very early pregnancy, which is more pronounced when certain foods are eaten.

Whatever the cause of cravings—and the jury is still out on this one—so long as you are meeting all of your daily needs with a healthy diet, there is no reason why you should not indulge your desire for the occasional treat.

The danger comes, of course, when your urge to satisfy a craving means that you are drawn to unhealthful items, such as coffee, alcohol, or cigarettes, which can harm your baby. Cravings of this nature should be ignored or curtailed. Otherwise, in moderation, enjoy whatever it is that you crave!

A craving for a nonfood item, such as coal, soap, or toothpaste, is known as "pica." On very rare occasions, pica can be a sign of more serious underlying problems, such as nutritional deficiency or psychological problems.

greenfile

If you crave cheese or ice cream, your body could be telling you that it needs more calcium. In fact, the unusual but not uncommon pregnancy craving of pickles and ice cream is not so hard to understand when you realize that vinegary foods (the pickles) help the body to release calcium (from the ice cream) into the bloodstream—it's nature's way of helping!

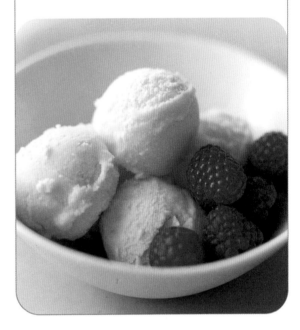

One of the most common taste dislikes in early pregnancy is toothpaste. Since commercial toothpastes contain fluoride, foaming agents, and other nasty chemicals, you can make your own.

Mix together 1 tablespoon baking soda, a pinch of salt, 1 teaspoon lemon juice, and 1 drop of peppermint essential oil, adding enough filtered water to mix the ingredients into a paste. The paste hardens if left open to the air, so store it in an airtight container. The beauty of your own homemade toothpaste is that you can choose any flavor you like—it doesn't have to be peppermint—and that way you are far less likely to have an aversion to cleaning your teeth.

Weight Gain

Weight is an emotive subject for women in the Western world. Many newly pregnant women are fearful of gaining excessive weight during the pregnancy that they will then have problems losing after the baby is born. In recognition of this Western obsession with being thin, many prenatal clinics have now ceased to weigh women at every visit, but naturally, many women still weigh themselves at home.

If you decide to keep a record of your weight gain at home, make sure you always use the same scale and that you always weigh yourself at the same time of day wearing just underwear, or similar clothing, each time.

Officially, the expected weight gain during pregnancy for a woman who is the appropriate weight for her height is between 24–35 lb (11–16 kg). However, if you are underweight at the start of your pregnancy, you could gain as much as 50 lb (22.7 kg) without cause for concern, although somewhere in the region of 28–40 lb (12.7–18 kg) is more common for thinner women. Conversely, if you are overweight when you conceive, you may not gain as much as the average expectation, but you should gain at least 15 lb (6.8 kg). A weight-gain range of 15–25 lb (7–11 kg) is anticipated if you are overweight.

It is unlikely that you will gain weight at a steady rate throughout the pregnancy—you tend to gain in fits and starts. Each woman's weight-gain pattern is unique to her. However, as a general rule of thumb, you can expect to gain moderately in the first trimester and at the beginning of the second trimester, say around 6–9 lb (3–4 kg) in the first 20 weeks. Thereafter, the rate of gain is faster—about 1 lb (450 g) per week on average.

> By week 32/33, you will be gaining weight faster than at any other time in your pregnancy. By week 37, your weight gain will probably be slowing down.

greenfile

It is a myth that smaller babies are easier to deliver. Studies show that an undernourished mother is more likely to deliver a baby who is also undernourished, and nutritionally deprived babies (low birth-weight infants) have a higher risk of newborn complications and delayed growth and development. So don't compromise your baby's health by trying to keep weight gain to a minimum.

What is more important than how much weight you gain is the rate of growth of your baby, and this is routinely monitored during prenatal care. You may find that your baby is growing rapidly in the later weeks of the pregnancy but that your weight gain actually slows down. So long as your baby is growing healthily, your emphasis should be on eating nutritiously and enjoying your food, rather than on how much weight you are putting on. You should try to consume about 2,000 calories of nutrient-rich foods a day, limiting calories from saturated fats and sugars.

Positive Body Image

Concerns about weight gain are often connected to how you view the pregnant form. If you think of yourself as a beached whale and unattractive while pregnant, you will probably consider any weight gain negatively. On the other hand, if you can view your body changes as beautiful and as a blessing, then you are more likely to have a positive approach to your new appearance and to the inevitable increase in your weight.

Even if you are unable to shake off a negative view of your pregnant body image, it is important that you do not consciously or unconsciously cut back on your food intake in an effort to keep your weight gain during pregnancy to a minimum. This is not a safe or sensible plan. Nor should you exercise excessively during pregnancy, particularly if the goal is minimizing weight gain.

Be reassured that most women are able to lose any excess weight after the birth of their baby through exercise and sensible eating. So don't be tempted to compromise a healthy pregnancy by dieting or excessive exercising.

Also, keep in mind that weight charts for expectant mothers, rather like those for growing babies, present ranges and averages. It doesn't mean you are unhealthy if you don't fit the right slot on the chart. However, if you are concerned at all by how much or how little weight you are putting on, speak to your prenatal care/obstetrical team.

BREAKDOWN OF AVERAGE PREGNANCY WEIGHT GAIN
Baby—7½ lb (3.4 kg)
Enlargement of uterus—2 lb (1 kg)
Placenta—1½ lb (750 g)
Amniotic fluid—2 lb (1 kg)
Breast enlargement—2 lb (1 kg)
Extra blood and fluid volume—8 lb (3.6 kg)
Extra fat stores—7 lb (3 kg)
Total—approx. 30 lb (14 kg)

If you are expecting twins, you can expect to gain an additional 10 lb (4.5 kg) over and above the average weight-gain guidelines.

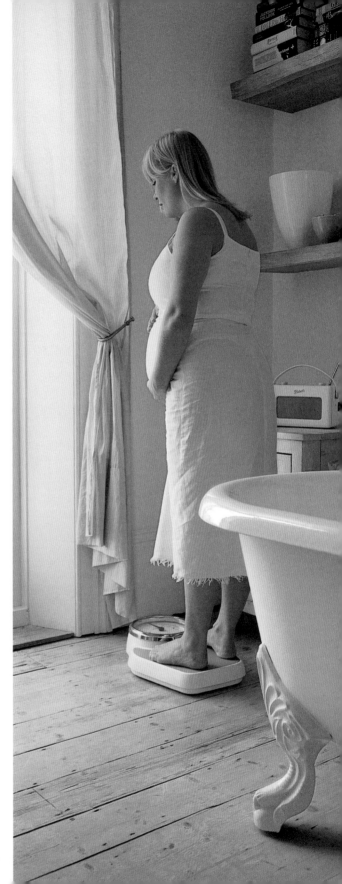

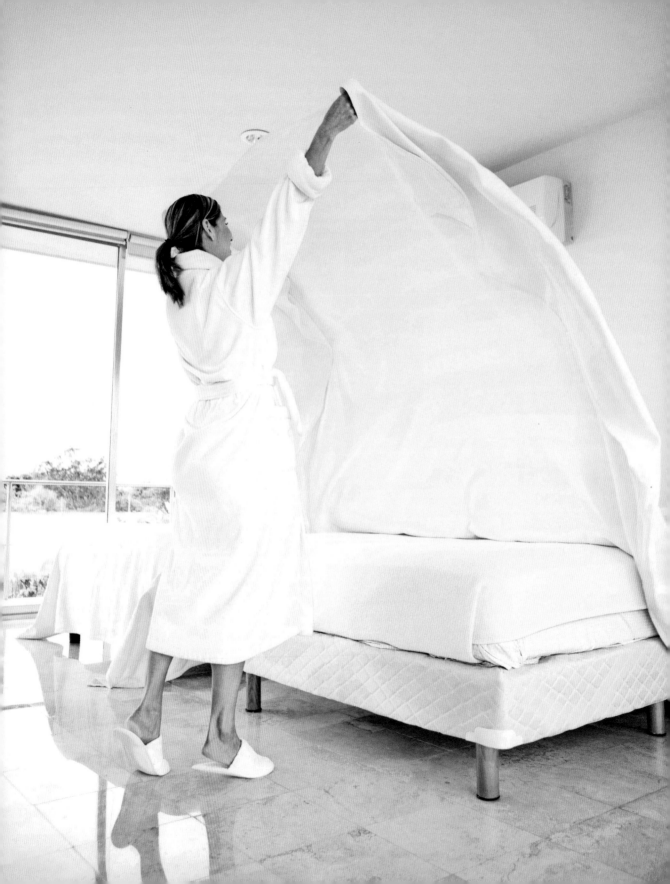

4 Healthy Living

The places where you live and work exert an unseen yet powerful influence on your life, both physically and emotionally. Most of the time, you give little thought to your living and working environment, but when you are pregnant, you are far more conscious about your surroundings and the effect they might have on you and your developing baby.

That's why this chapter draws your attention to the dangers that you might be exposed to in your home, especially when cleaning (see page 70), and there's advice on how to make the home and office environments safer, healthier, and greener (see page 75).

We also look at the environmental irritants, pollutants, and allergens that you may be exposed to, often through a busy social life, without necessarily realizing the risks these might pose. Certainly, when you read about the insidious dangers of secondhand smoke and over-the-counter medicines, you will understand the need for circumspection.

On a lighter note, this chapter will help you to indulge your natural "nesting" instinct with suggestions for a greener nursery (see page 76) and tips on how to choose the most attractive yet environmentally friendly and natural maternity wear and toiletries (see page 80).

Coping with Work

Unless you work in a hazardous environment or your work is physically strenuous, there is no reason why you shouldn't continue working throughout your pregnancy until around week 34, and a few women elect to work until their due date.

Nonetheless, there may be adjustments that you want to make to your normal work practices and working style for the sake of your health and general well-being.

Commuting

Commuting by bus or train shouldn't pose any particular problems, although you might like to consider changing your working hours to avoid the worst of the rush hour.

In the early stages of your pregnancy, morning sickness can make the early morning commute tricky. Try carrying ginger cookies, crackers, or a snack with you, or practise breathing exercises to alleviate the symptoms. If a bout of nausea persists, don't be afraid to get off the bus or train and wait until the nausea passes before reboarding—better to be late for work than sick on public transportation.

If you drive to work, try to avoid sitting in heavy traffic, and always close your car windows when going through a tunnel or in stationary traffic to avoid the buildup of fumes.

Even though it can be uncomfortable in the later stages of pregnancy, you should always wear a seatbelt in the car, whether you're driving or a passenger. The American Congress of Obstetricians and Gynecologists (ACOG) reports that research of crashes and safety belt use in pregnant women suggests that about four out of five babies would have been saved if their mothers had worn safety belts.

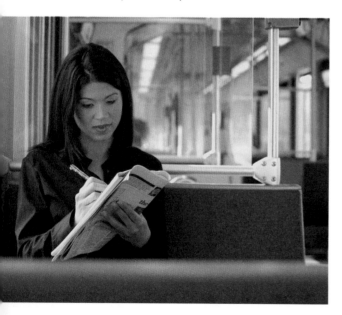

DRIVE SAFELY

For your safety and comfort, follow these rules when wearing your safety belt:

Always wear both the lap and shoulder belt.

Buckle the lap belt low on your hip bones, below your belly.

Place the shoulder belt off to the side of your belly and across the center of your chest (between your breasts). The upper part should cross your shoulder without chafing your neck.

Never place the shoulder belt under your arm, off your shoulder, or behind your back.

Make sure the belt fits snugly—belts worn too loosely or too high on the belly can cause broken ribs or injuries to your belly.

REMEMBER, most damage is caused when safety belts are not used at all.

greenfile

Some people believe that placing amber crystals, citrine, and tourmaline by the computer can offer some protection against electromagnetic fields and radiation.

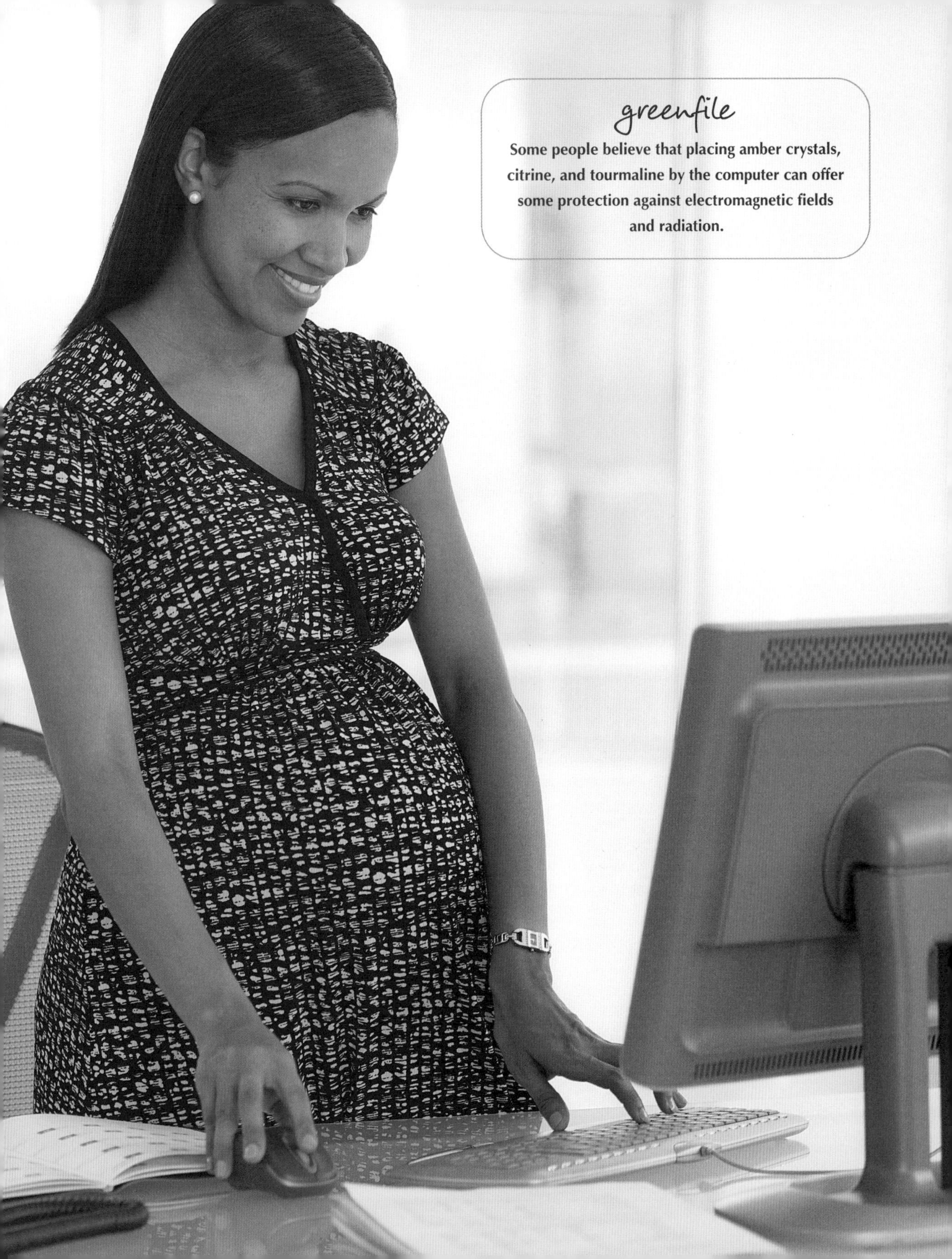

Computer Use

There's been speculation since the 1980s that computer monitors (also called video display units, or VDUs) are unsafe for pregnant women because of low levels of radiation (electromagnetic fields). However, in recent years, there have been many research studies into the subject, and there is no evidence that computer monitors cause any problems in unborn babies.

That said, this is completely counterintuitive for many women. In this case, you may prefer to use an anti-radiation, anti-static filter screen on your VDU for additional protection.

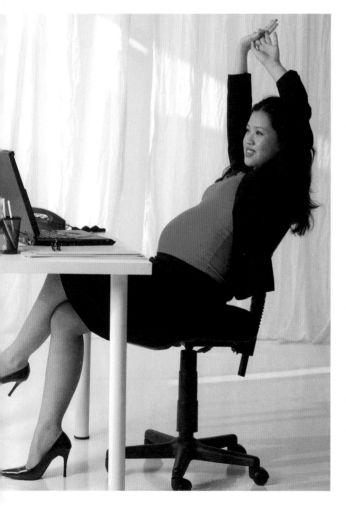

greenfile

The effects of positive ions produced by modern office technology, such as computers, can be neutralized by using an ionizer. Negative ions lead to improved mental alertness and health, whereas positive ions cause headaches, lethargy, tension, irritability, and discomfort.

What is inarguable is that sitting in front of the computer all day can strain your eyes, cause back pain, and make varicose veins worse. So be sure to take frequent breaks, walk around, and stretch your legs during the day.

Safety and Comfort

As an office worker, there are several precautions you can take to make sure you stay as healthy as possible while working throughout your pregnancy.

Don't be afraid to ask for or to accept help from your colleagues if you need it.

Reduce your exposure to stress at work. If you can't eliminate the stress factor (sadly, a difficult boss doesn't go away simply because you're pregnant), try to find ways to manage the stress, such as breathing exercises, visualization (see page 37), stretching, or simply taking a break and leaving the building. Physically removing yourself from the source of your stress can, on occasion, work wonders.

Take regular breaks throughout the working day. If you sit for long periods, then stand up and stretch. Conversely, if you've been standing, sit down and rest.

You must nourish yourself. Nutritious snacks and a proper lunch are essential—don't rely on the workplace vending machine and subsist on instant coffee, snacks, and cookies. It's important to stay hydrated, so drink plenty of water.

Keep the circulation flowing in your legs by putting your feet up when you take a break. A box, stool, or

WARNING Although working at a computer won't harm your developing baby, pregnant women are more susceptible to carpal tunnel syndrome (numb, achy fingers), so make sure you arrange your desk and chair at the optimum height.

another chair can make a perfectly adequate improvised footstool.

Dress in loose, comfortable clothing, and swap your killer heels for a lower heel or flat shoe (see page 80 for more advice on maternity wear).

Put a potted plant on your desk to bring good *yang* energy into your office.

Heavy Labor

You may have a job that requires you to perform considerable amounts of physical labor, which was fine before you were pregnant but could be a strain now. You need to speak to your employer if your job involves

- repetitive heavy lifting,
- pushing or pulling heavy loads,
- intense stair climbing,
- prolonged standing.

It may be possible to find a colleague who can take on some of the more dangerous aspects of your work; or you might be offered a temporary reassignment that is less physically demanding.

Alternatively, you may feel that you want to continue in the same post. In this case, to minimize the risks to you and your baby from physical exertion, you should take frequent breaks to rest and should monitor your physical and emotional stress levels closely.

Working with Chemicals

Should your job involve handling, transporting, or exposure to chemicals and pollutants on a daily basis, you may be best advised to speak to your employer about another temporary position or to stop working altogether, if this is economically feasible. This is because a number of chemicals and pollutants, in particular lead, mercury, carbon monoxide, pesticides, and anesthetics, have been shown to be particularly dangerous for both your own and your baby's health. Effects of exposure can include

- premature delivery,
- miscarriage,
- physical birth defects and deformitie,s
- developmental problems later in life.

Of course, it may be that you are unable to make other work arrangements. In which case, if you have to or choose to continue to work with chemicals, you are advised to follow strict safety precautions, namely

- wear protective clothing, such as gloves and a ventilator/mask, at all times,
- avoid direct contact with all chemicals,
- remove contaminated or soiled clothing as soon as possible,
- ask your employer to provide a risk assessment, information on health and safety hazards during pregnancy, and additional ventilation equipment.

AIR TRAVEL

Most of the time, the fact that your job involves lots of overseas travel is perhaps a huge attraction, but it can be a problem when you're pregnant. Many alternative health professionals advise against flying during the first trimester of pregnancy, especially if you have a history of miscarriage. This can be hard to explain if you haven't shared the news of your pregnancy with your boss or colleagues as yet.

If you have to travel by air for work, you might like to take the flower remedy yarrow, which can be beneficial but shouldn't be taken in the first trimester. Yarrow essence helps relieve queasiness and feelings of vulnerability, and protects you from absorbing environmental influences that are rife on a plane. There are also special travel sickness blends of flower essences available; but check that they are safe for use during pregnancy before buying.

A Clean, Green Home

As you already know, you are more susceptible to pollutants and chemicals when you're pregnant, so besides eliminating harmful substances from your diet and lifestyle, don't forget about the chemicals that you use every day around the house.

Many household cleaning products state on the packaging that they may not be safe for inhalation or use by pregnant women. Always read the labels carefully before using any cleaning product.

Since you are already introducing a more natural approach to health and diet into your lifestyle, why not take this opportunity to extend the green principle to keeping house as well?

Cleaning

Certainly, for the duration of your pregnancy, you should avoid the more potent commercial cleaners on the market. Nonetheless, even run-of-the-mill, perfumed proprietary brands can cause headaches, sneezing, sore throats, and irritated eyes, nose, and skin.

Your pregnancy is the perfect time to review your household cleaning products and opt for safer, greener alternatives that will ensure a healthier environment to bring your baby home to and in which your child can grow. Cut down on the number of products that you use, and avoid any that carry caution warnings or are corrosive or caustic.

A whole host of safer, milder, eco-friendly cleaners are now available in supermarkets and other stores. Based on natural cleansers, these products do actually work. Alternatively, why not use the proven ingredients that past generations used to clean the home? These everyday items are cheap and effective and they pose no health threat to you or your unborn child.

WARNING Keep all cleaning goods, whether commercial brands or natural products, out of the reach of inquisitive little fingers and mouths. Even natural or safer cleaners can pose a health risk when ingested.

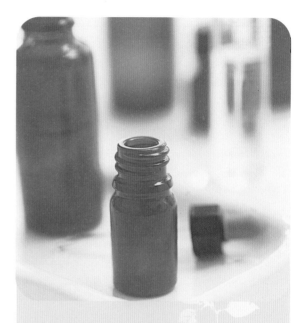

HOMEMADE CLEANING PRODUCTS
A mixture of ten drops of citrus or ylang-ylang oil in 2 quarts (2 liters) of water kills airborne bacteria and freshens the room.

One tablespoon of borax dissolved in about a quart (1 liter) of warm water cleans and deodorizes the fridge.

Baking soda mixed with water makes a natural cleaning cream that cuts through grease and dirt on most surfaces in the kitchen and bathroom.

Remove lime deposits from faucets by wrapping in a cloth soaked in white distilled vinegar. Leave for half an hour, then rinse clean.

To clean and deodorize drains, put 2 tablespoons of baking soda down the sink followed by half a cup of vinegar, leave for 20 minutes, then flush with cold water.

Natural Disinfectants

Instead of using store-bought disinfectants, try using certain herbal oils and extracts as a natural disinfectant in your home. The antifungal and antibacterial properties of oils, such as Australian tea tree oil, pine oil, and citrus seed extract, can be put to good use to wipe down nursery surfaces. However, they are not effective against harmful food bacteria, so do not rely on these in the kitchen or dining room.

Green Laundry

Try to reduce the amount of detergent you use in the form of washing liquids and powders, dishwashing liquids, and dishwasher products. Wherever possible, choose milder alternatives that are kinder to both the environment and your health. You should also opt for unscented, nonbiological varieties, which reduce the risks of allergic reactions.

You can cut your consumption of detergent powder by substituting baking soda for half the normal dose of commercial powder in each wash. For heavily soiled loads, add half a cup of borax to your usual detergent to boost its power, rather than using stronger detergents.

You can stop using fabric softeners completely, since their sole purpose is to coat clothing fibers

greenfile

Furniture polish containing sodium phosphate or turpentine can burn the skin and is dangerous when inhaled, especially during pregnancy. For an easy natural furniture polish, simply place 3 or 4 tea bags (black tea) in a large mug or bowl, and pour boiling water over. Allow to steep. When cool, remove the tea bags. Dip a cotton cloth into the tea and wipe over your wooden furniture. You don't even need to rinse. You'll be left with a lovely, natural sheen on your furniture.

greenfile

When replacing a washing machine or dishwasher, check out the eco-friendliness of your new appliance. Whenever possible, choose the greenest machine available at the right price.

temporarily, to prevent static cling: since your pregnancy clothes are probably made of natural fibers, such as cotton, wool, or linen, fabric conditioners are not necessary. If you still feel the need for fabric softeners, try adding one cup of white distilled vinegar to the dispenser drawer instead.

Green Thumbs

Pesticides, fertilizers, and herbicides all pose a health risk. While you are pregnant (and once you have a young family), it is well worth looking into the possibility of using organic and traditional gardening methods and integrated pest management. Both options are kinder to our environment and to you and your family.

Suggestions for a natural alternative to gardening pollutants include companion planting (plant three basil plants near a tomato plant to deter white flies and mosquitoes) and introducing pest-eating wildlife (a ladybug can eat more than 5,000 aphids per year) and natural barriers (slugs and snails dislike slithering over gritty surfaces, so surround precious plants with a thick sprinkling of crushed eggshells, pine needles, coffee grounds, or wood ash). Another option is to buy organic or chemical-free gardening products.

Air fresheners containing carbolic acid or formaldehyde can cause nausea. Use natural essential oils as air fresheners or freshly cut scented flowers, such as stocks.

WARNING Commercial toilet cleaners contain cresol, which is easily absorbed through the skin and can damage major organs. Instead, pour a quarter of a cup of borax around your toilet bowl and leave for an hour or overnight. Then flush for a clean, deodorized toilet.

Environmental Pollutants

Your surroundings can exert an unseen and occasionally dangerous influence on your health and that of your unborn baby. You can limit any health risks by organizing your home environment and changing certain lifestyle habits so that you and your baby enjoy the most natural well-being possible.

Smoking

Most research indicates that pregnant women should not smoke. When you smoke, your baby shares chemicals from the smoke you inhale. These chemicals adversely affect your baby's healthy growth and development. For example, carbon monoxide restricts your baby's oxygen supply, causing his heart to beat harder every time you smoke.

Recent studies also show that smoking during pregnancy can damage your baby's airways before he is even born. As a result, your child may develop smaller airways, making him more vulnerable to breathing problems, such as asthma, once he is born and as he grows up.

As well as all the well-documented threats to your health as a smoker, including a heightened risk of cancer, lung disease, and heart disease, there is a more immediate and dangerous risk to your health if you smoke when pregnant. Smoking can damage the placenta, leading to pregnancy complications, such as bleeding and placenta abruption (the placenta starts to come away from the uterus), and these complications can be life threatening for both you and your baby.

> ### STARTLING STATISTICS FOR PREGNANT SMOKERS
>
> Smokers are more likely to deliver babies prematurely and at a much lower birth weight.
>
> Smokers are five times more likely than nonsmokers to develop eclampsia, which is a leading cause of maternal deaths.
>
> Smokers are at greater risk of miscarriage and stillbirth.

The consensus is that you should give up smoking for the duration of your pregnancy at the very least. Quitting smoking might feel difficult, especially if you are already under stress, but you're not on your own—a great deal of support is available to you in the form of helplines (see Useful Contacts, page 156) and your primary care provider or obstetrician. When you see the drastic improvements to your life and health, and you know it is safeguarding your developing baby, it is really motivating.

Recreational Drugs

While you are pregnant, or if you are trying for a baby, you should avoid all recreational drug use.

Marijuana has not been conclusively proven to cause birth defects, but studies into its use during pregnancy have highlighted a link between the drug and growth and development problems, and low birth weights. Babies exposed to marijuana while they're in the womb are also more likely to be restless, irritable, and jumpy during the first few weeks after being born.

> ### greenfile
>
> Acupuncture (see page 108), when used by itself or in conjunction with other therapies, can be extremely beneficial in removing the craving for nicotine and so helping you to give up smoking. The acupuncture can be general or auricular (needles are inserted in specific parts of the ear).

PASSIVE SMOKING

It is definitely a step in the right direction for you to give up smoking, but if you still live or work with a smoker or spend time in a smoky atmosphere, you and your developing baby are still at grave risk from secondhand smoke.

Secondhand smoke, or Environmental Tobacco Smoke (ETS), as it is sometimes known, comes from the tip of a cigarette and the smoke that is breathed back out by the smoker. Wherever people smoke, there is secondhand smoke in the air, although you might not notice it because it is almost invisible and odorless.

Even if you open a window, secondhand smoke will still be present in a room after two and a half hours, despite the fact that you may not be able to see or smell it. Traveling with a smoker in a car is even worse, because all of the smoke is concentrated into a small space.

People that breathe secondhand smoke are at risk of the same diseases as smokers, including cancer and heart disease, because secondhand smoke contains 4,000 toxic chemicals. It is estimated that secondhand smoke causes thousands of deaths each year. And the dangers are far worse for pregnant women because, as we have seen, the toxins from inhaled smoke can cross the placenta and adversely affect your developing baby.

It is also worth thinking ahead: children are particularly affected by secondhand smoke because their bodies are still developing, and more than half of all American under-five children are growing up in homes where at least one parent is a smoker.

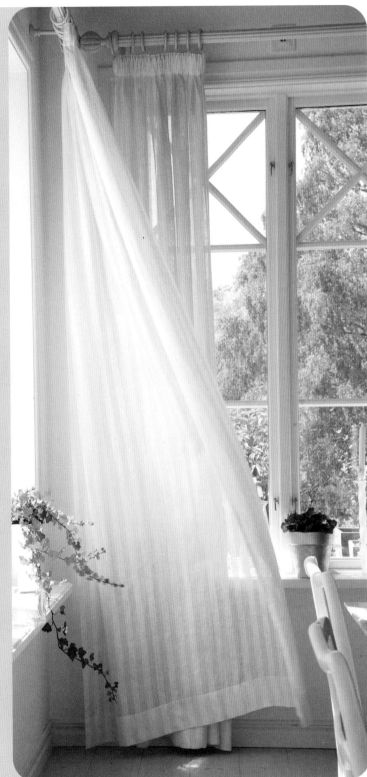

If marijuana is smoked with tobacco, additionally, the smoke causes the same problems as for cigarette smokers (see above).

Ecstasy According to recent research, taking ecstasy during pregnancy increases the risk of your baby's being born with abnormalities. In particular, babies had limb and heart problems, such as club foot and problems with bones and muscles. The drug poses risks at any time, but particularly during the first trimester, when a baby is going through the crucial early stages of development.

Cocaine and opiates are among the most dangerous recreational drugs for pregnant women, causing potentially life-threatening and long-lasting consequences for your baby.

For example, cocaine users are:

- Twice as likely as other women to give birth prematurely; and cocaine can cross the placenta and enter the circulation system of your baby
- At increased risk of miscarriage in the early stages of pregnancy
- At increased risk of premature labor during the later stages of pregnancy
- At increased risk of placental abruption, with all its inherent dangers

The babies of pregnant cocaine users are:

- At risk of permanent, serious brain damage
- Prone to a range of other abnormalities, including problems with the skull, heart, face, eyes, limbs, genitals, and intestines
- At risk of a range of permanent disabilities
- Likely to have a low birth weight

Heroin is another drug that can cause a host of problems for babies. In particular, it is linked with growth difficulties, stillbirth, and premature birth. In fact, half of all babies born to women who take heroin regularly arrive early. In addition, heroin can be passed to a baby through breast milk, and babies may be born suffering with withdrawal from heroin, showing symptoms, such as irritability, restlessness, distress, and feeding difficulties.

Of course, if you have a recreational drug problem, no one is underestimating how hard it is to stop its use, but there is help available (see Useful Contacts, page 156). The dangers to your unborn child of continued drug use are too serious to ignore.

Prescription Medications

As soon as you realize that you are pregnant, you should consult your doctor about the safety of any prescribed medications that you are taking. Some are able to cross the placenta and adversely affect your baby. However, you should not abruptly stop taking medication without first seeking advice.

Some over-the-counter medications (OTC) can also affect or harm the fetus or baby, so you should consult your pharmacist before taking any OTC medicine. OTC medication labels should be checked, because they contain warnings against use during pregnancy and breast-feeding, if applicable.

Certain types of drugs are particularly problematic. They include antihistamines (commonly contained in cough and cold remedies, allergy drugs, motion sickness drugs, and sleep aids) and nonsteroidal anti-inflammatory drugs (NSAIDs). Examples of nonprescription NSAIDs are aspirin, ibuprofen (e.g. Brufen), naproxen sodium, diclofenac, and ketoprofen, although they may be marketed under a variety of different brand names. NSAIDs should not be

greenfile

Do not attempt to give up drugs or deal with addiction alone. Get help from a specialist, a support group such as Narcotics Anonymous, or a complementary medical practitioner.

WARNING If your pregnancy is unplanned and you've been taking drugs, you should stop doing so as soon as possible, as the early stages of development in the womb are crucial, and your baby may have been exposed to harm.

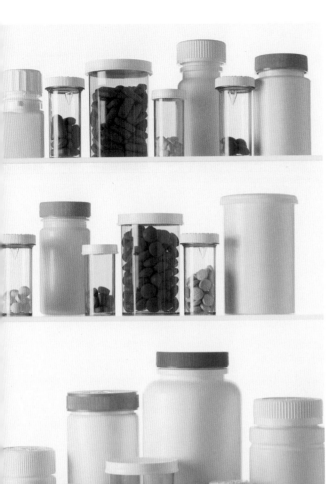

Why not take the following precautions to minimize the risk to you and your baby of any environmental pollutants:

Diagnostic X-rays are dangerous for your baby. Wherever possible, postpone unnecessary X-rays or CT scans until after your baby is born. If an X-ray is necessary, tell the doctor or radiologist that you're pregnant, and make sure you're given a protective lead apron to wear.

Don't stand directly in front of a microwave oven while it's in use.

Avoid chemical hazards, such as cleaning agents and garden pesticides (see A Clean, Green Home, page 70).

Radon, a naturally occurring, radioactive gas, can cause cancer. The Environmental Protection Agency (EPA) advises pregnant women to contact their local government or ecological group to establish whether they live in a radon-contaminated area. Alternatively, you could buy a radon detector to monitor radon levels in your home.

Avoid using aluminum or copper cookware, and don't wrap food in aluminum foil.

Although there is no scientific evidence to suggest that an electric blanket or heating pad can harm your fetus, it is commonly believed that you should avoid sleeping with one on.

The risk of domestic carbon monoxide poisoning caused by leaks from faulty furnaces, wood-burning stoves, fireplaces, gas heaters, gas stoves and space heaters can be prevented by early detection with the use of household carbon monoxide detectors and by having these items regularly serviced.

In the United States, you can ask your local environmental safety office to test the lead levels in your drinking water. In Britain, your water company will tell you how likely it is that there are high lead levels in your drinking water. If you are concerned, contact your water company; a representative should take a sample from your home, if necessary, and the company should tell you the results.

used during the last three months of pregnancy unless specified by a doctor, because they may cause problems for your baby or complications during delivery.

As a general rule, avoid all medication during your pregnancy unless it is specifically prescribed for you. Instead, look at a number of natural alternatives that can help with most of the common ailments (see Chapter 7, Health & Well-being). However, a word of caution: just because something is natural does not mean it's not potent. Get advice before using any herbal or complementary medicines.

Preparing the Nursery

It is a natural instinct, especially in the latter months of your pregnancy, to nest build. Preparing the nursery for your new baby can be a source of much delight. But, without wishing to dampen your enthusiasm, it is important that you bear a few safety factors in mind.

When you are pregnant, you and your unborn child are vulnerable to environmental irritants, allergens, and toxins; so, when assembling your new nursery, you want to take every precaution to protect the both of you.

The good news is that in the past few years a much greater choice of green, environmentally friendly, and safe products with which to decorate and furnish your nursery has appeared on the market. They pose far fewer, if any, health risks than synthetic equivalents.

Decorating

You should never sand or repaint your baby's room (or any other room) when pregnant. In old houses, sanding can disturb old lead paint, creating a toxic dust, which you then breathe in. It is widely known that lead can cross the placenta, so not only could this dust give you lead poisoning; it could also harm your unborn child.

Lead poisoning is such a serious condition that if your partner works with old paint, or takes on the decorating himself, avoid him until he has showered and replaced his work clothes.

If you are concerned about the potential presence of lead, there are commercial companies who will come into your home and test walls, windowsills, doorjambs, and house dust. If unacceptable levels are found—or even traces, for that matter—the company is equipped and qualified to remove the paint safely. Alternatively, you can get a self-test kit from home centers to check whether your paintwork contains lead; but it will not tell you in what quantity.

If professional removal is not possible, apply a fresh coat of nontoxic paint over the old paint, but be careful that it does not start to chip or get repeatedly rubbed, because this could release lead from the old paint layers underneath.

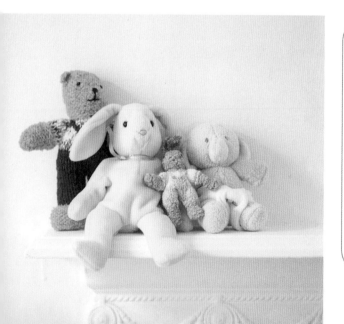

greenfile

Whichever paint you choose, it is important to air the nursery well before your baby is moved into the room. In fact, in Chinese tradition, it is recommended that you air all rooms and replace stale energy once a day by opening windows and encouraging a through draft.

Don't be tempted to use an air freshener to do the job of airing the room. These often contain carbolic acid or formaldehyde, which can cause nausea in pregnant women.

Choosing Paint

When choosing a paint or wood finish, check the label for levels of volatile organic compounds (VOCs), which readily vaporize into the air we breathe. Their effects have been linked to headaches, nausea, dizziness, nerve damage, and, in extreme cases, to liver and kidney disease. They are also suspected carcinogens. Low-VOC or VOC-free paints are now readily available in home centers.

For a green option, you can choose from a wide range of eco-friendly paints and natural varnishes available from specialist and online distributors. These healthier alternatives to conventional paints include organic, milk (casein), water-based, and natural types. They use primarily natural solvents, such as citrus and other plant oils, and are free of preservatives and biocides. They tend to be more expensive than synthetic paints and often require more care and effort to mix and apply.

Lead-based paint has been banned in most Western countries for many years, but don't underestimate the danger from old and chipped lead paint in older properties. Never dry- or power-sand old paint. Lead poisoning is less likely if old paint is treated with a damp waterproof abrasive paper or with chemical stripper.

Choosing Floor Coverings

Expectant parents often decide to lay a new carpet in a baby's nursery, as this is considered to be most hygienic. If you choose this option, make sure it is laid

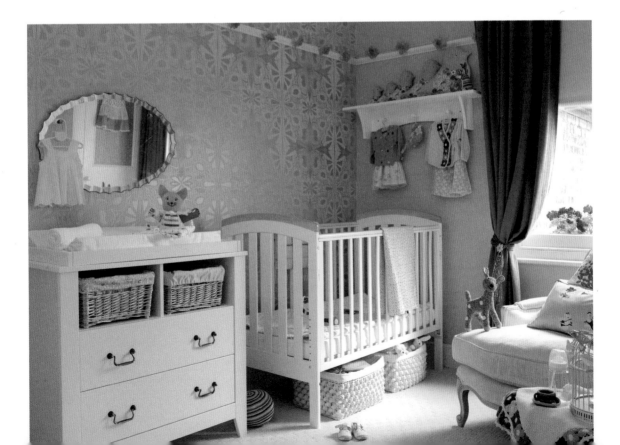

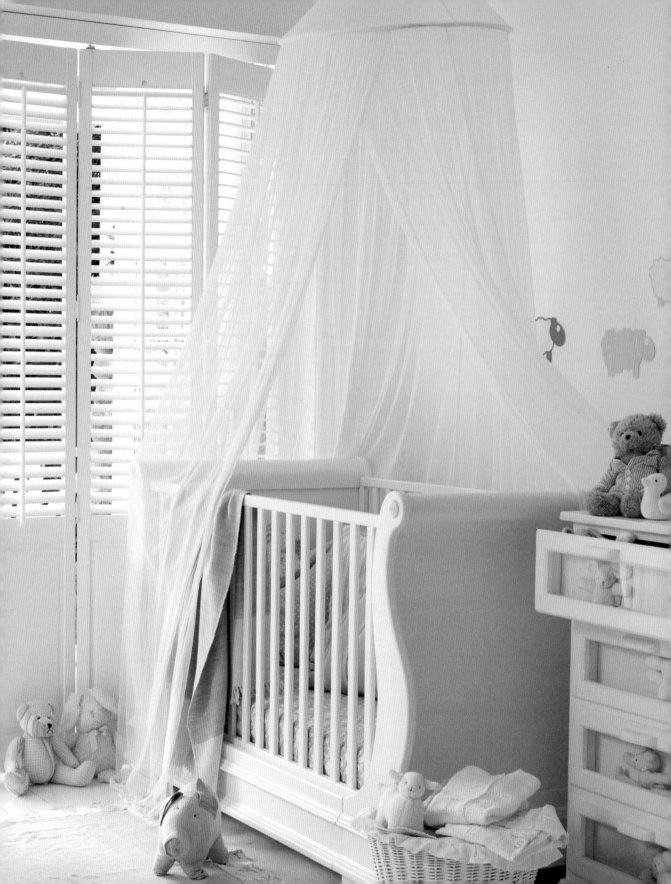

greenfile

Tack down the carpet, rather than gluing because the adhesives used for carpet laying are high in VOCs and give off toxic fumes.

If there is a history of allergies or asthma in the family, you may be best advised to avoid wall-to-wall carpeting in the baby's room, since it is believed that the dust mites that live in carpet pile worsen allergic conditions.

Fill your home with houseplants, which absorb carbon dioxide in the air while adding oxygen. Not only are indoor plants really attractive, but they're good for you all. Any of the common houseplants, such as African violets, spider plants, wandering Jew, prayer plants, Boston ferns, and umbrella plants, are perfectly safe. Avoid oleander and lilies, which can be toxic.

at least a couple of months before the baby is going to use the room, because new synthetic carpets give off toxic fumes for quite some time after installation. By the same token, make sure you are not in the house while the carpet is being laid, and get your partner or a friend to air the room well before you enter or spend any time in there.

A better option is to stick with natural-fiber carpets, such as wool, but these cost considerably more than their synthetic counterparts, and some may still have synthetic backings.

If you prefer to clean the existing carpet, use topical treatments, such as anti-dust mite sprays (having first checked the packaging to make sure that they are safe to use when pregnant), and a vacuum cleaner with a fine-particle-trapping filter to control allergens. To deodorize carpets naturally, sprinkle with baking soda, leave for an hour, then vacuum.

Choosing Soft Furnishings

There are so many beautiful fabrics to choose from when furnishing a nursery—gorgeous quilts, sheets, blankets, crib bumpers, curtains. When trying to find the perfect choices for your nursery, bear in mind that it makes best environmental sense to choose natural and untreated fabrics.

If you choose synthetic fabrics for curtains, the heat and light coming through the window will cause the fibers to break down and give off gases into the room, which could be detrimental to you and to your baby

once he is sleeping there. Natural fabrics, such as cotton, linen, and hemp, are the best choices for nursery curtains.

Blinds make suitable, nonallergenic alternatives to curtains. Whether the blind is made from steel, wood, bamboo, or aluminum, make sure it has not been chemically finished. If it has, allow it to aerate well away from you for a few days before installing.

Finally, it is worth bearing in mind that whereas these environmental considerations are important when decorating and furnishing your baby's first room, you should not worry about them to the extent that it detracts from the pleasure of preparing the room. Planning the nursery should be a joy, not a concern. Buying healthful and environmentally friendly decorating and furnishing options is obviously the best choice for optimum health for you and your baby, but even if you implement just some of these recommendations, that is a step in the right direction.

greenfile

As you prepare to welcome a new baby into your home, find time to sort out your house, not just the nursery. De-clutter and create space for you and your new baby, both literally and metaphorically. Keep the nursery clear and light, and spray the room with water containing a few drops of essential oil of mandarin or grapefruit.

Maternity Wear and Toiletries

No longer do pregnant women have to rely on wearing baggy, shapeless clothing to accommodate their bump. Now an impressive range of maternity clothes is available for both leisure and business wear, with many department stores and boutiques offering ranges for moms-to-be. Better yet, there are increasing numbers of outlets that stock or specialize in eco-friendly, organic maternity clothing, which is great news for green expectant moms.

Having said that, remember that the length of time when maternity clothes are a necessity is short. The best green option (best for your wallet also) would be to buy just a few "core" outfits, then borrow most of your maternity wardrobe from a friend. If she doesn't want it back, you might pass it on to another pregnant friend when you've finished with it.

Bear in mind that your body temperature will increase with pregnancy, so you should favor clothes made from natural fibers, preferably organic and undyed or untreated cotton or wool, silk, and cashmere. Unlike synthetics, natural fibers breathe and are less chafing.

When the weather turns cold, dress in layers that will draw the sweat away from your body—you can peel off or add layers as you please to regulate your temperature.

With the right clothing, you will feel more confident about your appearance and good about yourself.

Proper Support

When you are pregnant, your bra size can vary from two to four sizes larger. The increase in weight and size of the breasts during pregnancy will cause the skin to stretch and the breasts to drop, which is why it is important for pregnant women, however big or small your breasts, to be fitted for a new bra regularly (every couple of months). It is probably worth investing in some good maternity pants and pantyhose, too, especially toward the end of your pregnancy. Not only are these extremely comfortable, because they fit above your bump, but they also help to prevent varicose or spider veins and other leg problems.

greenfile

An ingenious clothing device that will extend the wear of your ordinary wardrobe well into your pregnancy is the pregnant tummy tube. It is a piece of stretchy fabric in a loop that supports your bump while also holding up your unbuttoned pants and maintaining a stylish look. There are plenty to choose from, but look for those made of an environmentally sustainable material, such as bamboo.

Of course, your mother's solution to the same problem was an ever-lengthening elastic band threaded through the buttonhole and looped around the button of your pants, coupled with a smock!

DRY CLEANING

If you use a dry cleaner, ask if they use perc (perchloroethylene), benzene, sulfuric acid, or toluene—chemicals that at high levels can cause headaches and faintness. Dry-cleaned clothes not exposed to these chemicals are safer.

When you pick up your clothes from the dry cleaners, make sure you ventilate them well, preferably outdoors, before wearing them.

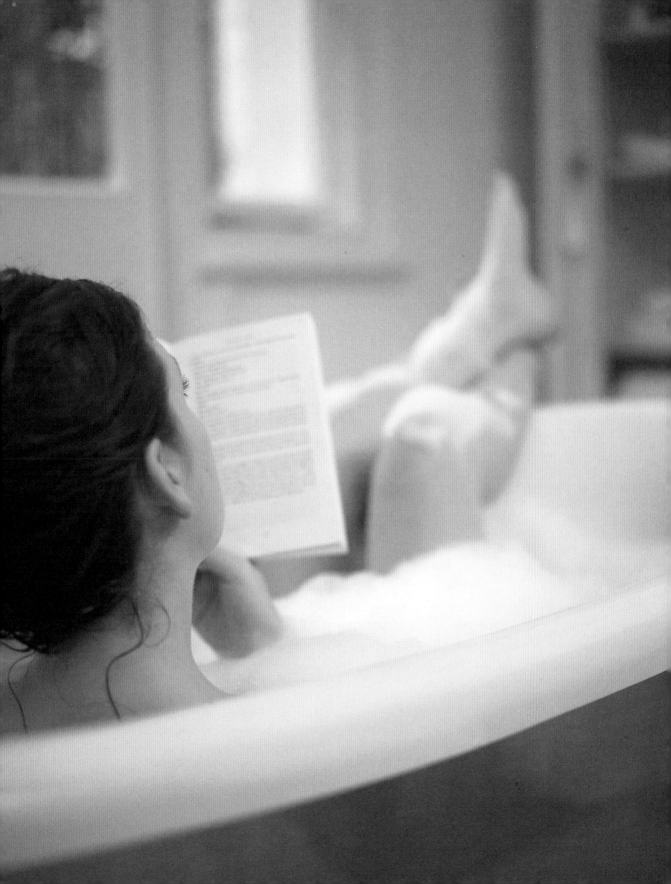

Cosmetics and Toiletries

Now is the time to take special care of your skin and to pamper yourself a little. Many women seem to get a wonderful "pregnancy glow" to their complexion, while others suddenly develop bad skin for the first time in their lives. Similarly, some unfortunate women suffer from stretch marks while others get away without so much as a blemish. How your skin reacts to pregnancy is something of a lottery. However, if you feed and treat your skin with natural products, rather than off-the-shelf cosmetics and toiletries that contain countless chemicals, you stand a better chance of continuing to have healthy, vibrant skin throughout your pregnancy.

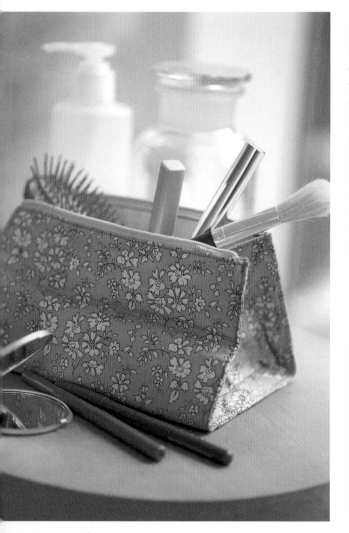

Skincare

There are so many lovely, natural, and effective lotions and creams to keep your skin supple during your pregnancy that there is no need to choose conventional beauty products that contain parabens. These are a class of chemicals that are used as preservatives in cosmetics and toiletries. They are a cause of particular concern because you leave these products on your skin for a long time, so increasing exposure time. Some studies have linked the estrogen-like effects of parabens to breast cancer and reproductive abnormalities, so it is well worth avoiding paraben-containing products in favor of organic or natural beauty products.

In fact, there is a plethora of small companies making a wonderful range of natural skincare lotions and creams especially for pregnant women. Always check out the list of ingredients used to assure yourself that their natural claims are authentic, and then treat yourself to a few items. If you would be happier rubbing only pure, unadulterated natural products into your skin, the following oils, creams, and unctions are recommended:

- vitamin E oil or lotion
- aloe vera gel
- wheatgerm or almond oil
- cocoa or shea butter
- calendula cream

greenfile

Antiperspirants containing aluminum chlorohydrate or/and aluminum zirconium chlorohydrate block skin pores and can cause inflammation. Choose a natural alternative containing ammonium alum or zinc ricinoleate, which are naturally occurring salts that will not cause any irritation and which "fix" sweaty smells.

Haircare

Many women find that their hair tends to dry out during pregnancy, so after washing with a natural, nontoxic shampoo, apply a natural conditioner. The following recipe is easy to make at home.

Peel one avocado and mash the flesh in a bowl. Add some coconut milk, a little at a time, while mashing with a fork. Keep blending until you reach the consistency of bottled conditioner. Apply by combing through the hair and leaving for 10–15 minutes before rinsing.

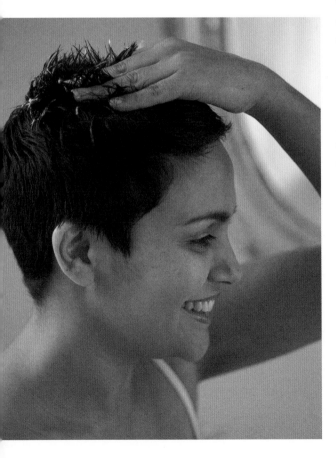

Dentalcare

Toothpastes containing ammonia, ethanol, formaldehyde, mineral oil, or saccharin should be avoided. Instead, choose baking soda, peppermint oil, or natural herb toothpastes.

Tooth and gum problems are common, especially in the first half of pregnancy. Instead of using a conventional mouthwash after brushing, steep a chamomile tea bag in freshly boiled water for 15 minutes. When cooled, rinse around the mouth, then spit out. (See also page 131.)

Nailcare

If you normally use nail polish on your fingernails or toenails, you may not realize that conventional nail polish is one of the most toxic of all beauty products, containing a mix of phthalates, formaldehyde, and a host of other VOCs (volatile organic compounds). And what with the acetone you need to remove old or chipping polish, you may wish to forgo a full manicure or pedicure while you're pregnant.

However, in the last few years, a variety of nontoxic nail polishes has appeared on the market. Some are water based and others use a natural mineral base but all are alleged to be toxin free. Nonetheless, even with these new polishes, it is worth taking the precaution of polishing your nails less frequently than usual; if you do so, make sure the room is well ventilated.

CAMPAIGN FOR SAFE COSMETICS

For more information on body and face care, check out the Campaign for Safe Cosmetics. They have a "Compact for Cosmetics," an agreement that more than 600 companies who fit the criteria for safe products have signed. See Useful Contacts, page 156, for site details if you want to check whether your favorite cosmetics company has signed, making the products we put on our face and body more healthful for us and our environment.

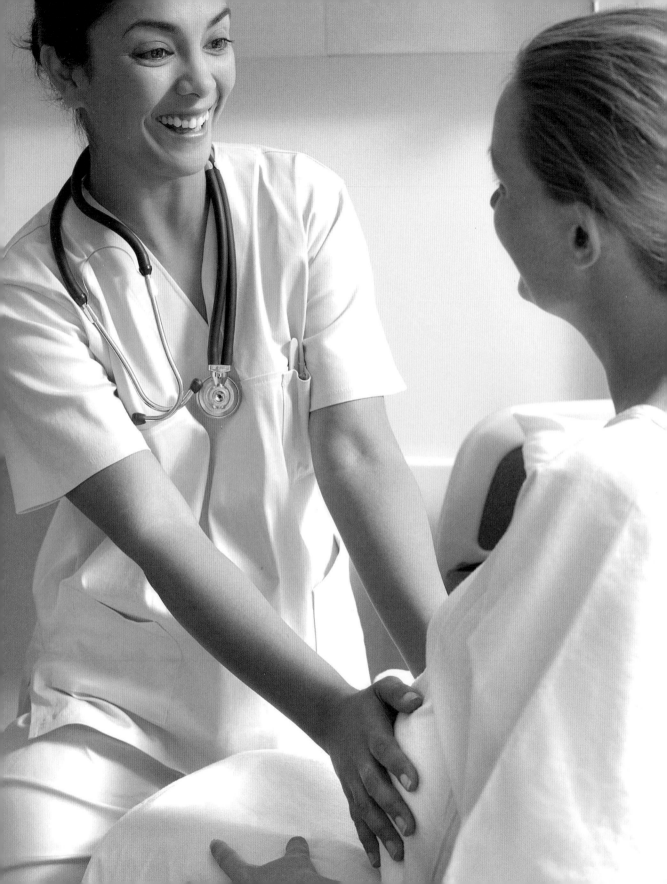

5 Prenatal Care

The first few weeks and months of pregnancy are so exciting; yet even as you are coming to terms with your news, you are faced with some early decisions that have to be made regarding what kind of pregnancy you would like, how you want to be cared for during this time, and what kind of birth you want for you and your baby.

There is a great deal of information available to you and a lot to digest in quite a short space of time. You may well have a clear idea of the overall approach you would like to take—and since you are reading this book, it is probably fair to assume that a natural approach to pregnancy would best suit you—but you might be hazy on detail.

It is well worth reading about what's available, both generally and in your locality, speaking to healthcare professionals and to other parents who have been through the experience personally, before you come to any firm decisions.

This chapter looks at choosing the care provision that best suits your inclinations and needs (see page 86) and the benefits of creating a birth plan (see page 89), and provides a review of the prenatal checkups (see page 92) and testing (see page 96) that are on offer.

Finally, why not think about joining a childbirth education class (page 98). There are classes to suit every taste, and some put more emphasis on a natural pregnancy and birth than others. In any case, classes can provide a great forum for you to explore all the issues about prenatal care and birth that interest you.

Choosing a Maternity Caregiver

Whom you choose to look after you during your pregnancy, and perhaps in labor too, will affect the type of experience you have and the care you receive. These prenatal professionals are responsible for your health and the health of your baby throughout your pregnancy and for the tone of your childbirth experience, so it is important to choose a team or individual who is not only qualified and competent but whom you can trust and feel comfortable with.

This section provides you with a general overview of the main types of care providers currently available in the United States. Since many offer a free consultation, you can decide which care provider offers the approach that you are looking for.

Prenatal Caregivers

Most practitioners, whether it be an obstetrician, certified nurse-midwife, or traditional midwife, will see you on roughly the same prenatal schedule of monthly and then bi-monthly visits until 36 weeks, when visits become weekly.

Direct-entry and Certified Professional Midwives (CPM) tend to believe that pregnancy and birth are natural processes and that they are at the birth to assist and guide you so that you can enjoy a healthy, natural experience. Direct-entry and certified professional midwives primarily attend home births, but many also provide prenatal and birthing services at birthing centers or clinics.

However, the right to give birth at home has been challenged in most states, and midwives are illegal in some states. Therefore, you may well meet opposition from other healthcare providers if you choose to have a home birth attended by a CPM.

A **Nurse-Midwife** has completed the same training as a registered nurse but s/he then specializes in midwifery. A nurse-midwife is a good choice if you are seeking medical care that puts the emphasis on the woman. Some nurse-midwives may even support the use of complementary and alternative practices during the birth. Nonetheless, the decisions taken by a nurse-midwife must reflect the protocols and stance of their supervisory obstetrician and the hospital or birthing center where they practise.

Finally, an **obstetrician** is a trained physician who then studies for an additional four years in obstetrics and gynecology. Most obstetricians rely on technology for your prenatal care and birth experience, although your views and preferences should be taken into account. Occasionally, a hospital may provide an **Osteopathic Obstetrician** on the staff. These are trained osteopathic physicians who have a specialty in obstetrics. Although they have undergone the same training as obstetricians and are able to perform cesarean sections and other surgery, because osteopathic training generally integrates an acceptance of holistic therapies alongside allopathic medicine, many osteopathic obstetricians are more open to a natural approach to childbirth.

Hospital Births

Some women feel reassured by having medical back-up close to hand, especially for a first baby. Others know that they will need medical intervention.

> Most obstetricians are men but this is changing and the rate of female medical residents is now around 50 percent.

HOME BIRTH

If you are a healthy woman with a normal pregnancy and a loving home environment, then a home birth is as safe as a hospital birth—and it is possible, whether this is your first or your fifth baby.

That said, there are very, very few American women who go for this option, despite increased publicity and popularity as a result of the Hollywood move toward home births by celebrity moms such as Cindy Crawford, Pamela Anderson, and Demi Moore.

For historical and political reasons, doctors no longer offer their services at home births or very rarely, so your primary attendant at a home birth is likely to be a midwife. Each state has its own legislation regarding qualifications required, so check with your doctor or healthcare provider.

Although you can follow whichever philosophy you want for your own home birth, it still needs planning and careful consideration. However, most midwives and doctors can advise on items to have at hand, etc.

If you are not sure whether you would prefer a home birth, you might find it helpful to talk to other people who have had home births in your area. They can tell you how easy or difficult it is to arrange a home birth there, and direct you toward any particularly helpful midwives. Talking to other people who have given birth at home can be a great confidence boost—it helps to know that there are other women, just like you, who have done it.

greenfile

Some, but not all, hospitals and birth centers are now equipped with birth pools for labor. However, they cannot be booked and are available strictly on a "first come, first served" basis. Some hospitals will allow you to bring a hired birth pool in with you but, again, not all. Check your hospital or birth center's stance on water births, whether they have midwives who are trained in water births, and how many women have had a water birth in recent months.

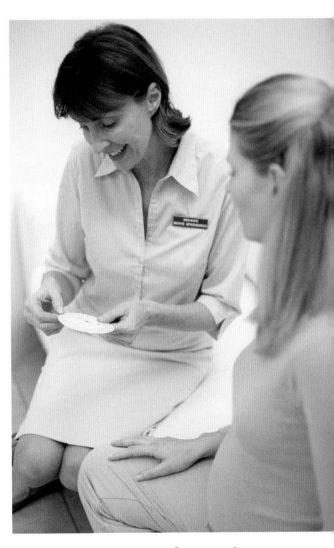

In either case, the obvious choice is to book your birth in an obstetric/maternity unit of a hospital.

Although most hospitals have worked hard to improve the birthing environment and to respect the wishes of pregnant women, many still see birth as a medical event rather than a natural process. You can, therefore, expect to undergo a number of routine protocols and procedures.

In order to decide which hospital is most likely to give you the birth experience you desire—and it is not impossible to have a holistic birth within a hospital environment—you should take the labor and delivery tours that are on offer to expectant mothers and their partners. Here you will pick up on the hospital's ethos and approach, and this can be clarified when you speak to your doctor or midwife.

Birth center

Birth centers offer facilities with homelike surroundings and low-level medical equipment for low-risk births. There are three different varieties of birth center: independent, freestanding facilities; hospital-linked facilities that are near a maternity department; and facilities that are housed within a hospital yet are treated as a separate service. You might expect a home-style, private room equipped with queen or full beds, comfortable chairs, and even a kitchen.

Both doctors and midwives are in attendance at a birth center and you can expect a less medically-centered approach to the birth. Most birth centers discharge you with your baby within 6–12 hours of the the birth, with additional postnatal visits at home.

This option holds much appeal for mothers who want a more natural, non-intervention birth but who do not feel confident about a home birth. However, it is not an option that is available to you if your pregnancy has been classified as high risk. If you are unaware of the risk factor associated with your pregnancy and birth, talk to your practitioner. Another obstacle to having your baby at a birth center is the fact that many are only open to certain doctors or midwives. Potentially, your midwife or physician may not be allowed to bring clients to your chosen birth center, so it is worth checking this early on in your pregnancy.

greenfile

Evidence suggests that when care is midwife-led and birth takes place outside a consultant unit, intervention rates are lower. Moreover, studies show that babies born in birth centers find it easier to establish breastfeeding

greenfile

The Coalition for Improving Maternity Services (CIMS) comprises international organizations and individuals who promote the best care and well-being of mothers and babies. They have a system of rating hospitals, birth centers, and home birth services depending on how mother-friendly they are. They also have an online birth survey so that you can share your experiences with other women and learn in advance about the experiences of others regarding your local services.

For more details, see the CIMS website (see Useful Contacts, pages 156–157).

The American Journal of Public Health published a study which compared birth outcomes from various venues. According to the study, the Farm Midwifery Center in Tennessee, which assists mothers wanting a home birth experience, reported use of forceps, vacuum extractors, or cesarean sections in 2 percent of births compared to a rate of 27 percent for the same procedures in comparative hospitals.

In 2006, the rate of home births in the USA was 0.59 percent of all births. This rate is comparable to that in other industrialized countries, but with two notable exceptions: England has experienced a rise in its home birth rate from 1.0 percent in 1989 to 2.7 percent in 2006, while the Netherlands has maintained astonishing rates of home birth of approximately 30 percent.

Birth Plans

For those of you who are not familiar with the concept, a birth plan is a written outline of what you would ideally like to happen at your baby's birth. It's an opportunity to reiterate the things that are important to you. Your doctor or midwife will have it on hand at the birth to check what has been discussed and agreed with you during your pregnancy.

Whether or not you adhere strictly to your birth plan, its principal benefit is that it serves to focus your mind. In order to write a plan, you have to give serious consideration to the type of birth experience that you would most like and what this might involve. For example, do you want a hospital or home birth? What kind of pain relief would you prefer, if any? Whom do you want with you at the birth? Do you want any specialist equipment, such as a birthing pool or stool? And how would you like to welcome your newborn into the world?

To answer these questions, you must naturally rely on your intuition and personal preferences, but you must also be well informed. And, to that end, writing a birth plan can prompt you to seek out reliable information and to ask pertinent questions of your doctor and other health professionals. You might also like to speak to friends who have recently had babies and get the benefit of their experiences.

Considerations

Clarity Bear in mind that the way you present the information in your birth plan can be just as important as the facts themselves. For example, you stand a better chance of ensuring that your wishes are met if you keep the contents concise, clear, and easy to read. You should also be as precise as possible in stating what you want.

Flexibility Many women who have set their heart on a certain style of delivery feel frustrated and disappointed when the birth does not go according to plan. Yet you should not feel that you have failed if you have not stuck exactly to your birth plan. The most

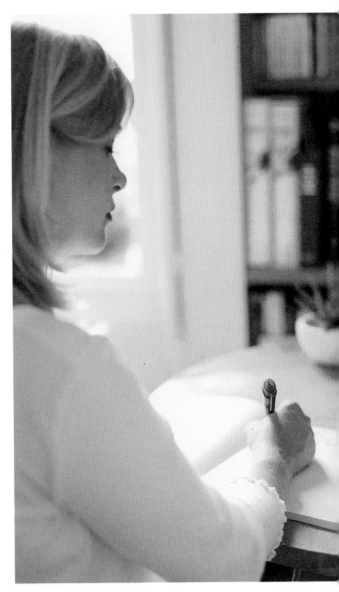

important advice to remember is to keep an open mind. Nobody can know how they are going to feel in labor until they get there. That's true even of women who have had babies before.

Experts agree that a birth plan is most effective if you remain flexible and recognize that it is a guideline rather than a bible. This approach avoids disappointment if events beyond your control mean your plans have to change, and it also allows for the fact that you may feel very different on the day. Staying open-minded gives you greater choice.

Healthcare conventions What is harder to accept is if the element of choice is removed. It may happen that you want to stick to your birth plan but this is made difficult, not for health reasons, but because of resistance from professionals involved in the birth or because of protocol. Occasionally, women report feeling that the hospital had let them down by not giving them the experience they wanted, despite assurances during their prenatal care.

Most hospitals now are far more accommodating of women who wish to have a natural or intimate birth experience—but not all. If your birth plan comprises anything that might be considered unconventional—for example,

• dimming of lights in the delivery room
• playing of relaxing music
• use of birthing pools, stools, or other birthing aids
• resistance to electronic monitoring
• resistance to artificial rupture of membranes
• delivery while standing or kneeling

—you are best advised to discuss your wishes well in advance with the hospital.

Another way to improve the chances of compliance with your wishes is to include a statement in your birth plan saying, "Do not perform the following without my express permission." Then to list the procedures over which you would like to be consulted.

A birth plan can bolster your resolve and give you the confidence to know your "starting" position. You then have to be convinced of the case to take a different course of action.

Partner support It can also be useful to get your birth partner involved in dialogue and decision making, since you may not be thinking clearly during labor. He (or she) can talk to staff and then talk to you. A birth partner should remain calm, think clearly, and hopefully champion your case.

In most cases, it never comes to this; and the birth plan is simply a useful tool to help you make certain decisions about the birth of your baby. Some prenatal notes even include a page for a birth plan. In general, it's perfectly acceptable to midwives, but not all women want to put their wishes down in writing; They prefer to wait and see what happens—and that's fine, too.

Things to Think About: Labor

Birth partners Research shows that it's helpful to have someone, such as a partner, friend, or relative, with you during your labor.

Carers Student midwives and medical students have to attend births as part of their training. Are you happy for students to be present?

Breaking your waters In some hospitals, the practice is to "break the waters" to speed up labor. Do you agree to having your waters broken artificially (see pages 143–4)?

Being induced Discuss with your obstetrician or midwife whether you want to be induced or not and what methods are available (see page 144).

Pain relief What's your position on self-help, such as moving around, changing positions, breathing techniques, relaxing in a bath, or massage? Do you have a view on Entonox (gas and air), TENS, pethidine, or epidural? Is there a form of pain relief you definitely do not want to try (see page 147)?

Fetal monitoring Your doctor listens to the baby's heartbeat to detect any signs of distress. S/he may use a hand-held device or an electronic monitor, which can impede movement. In some hospitals, electronic monitoring is routine. What's the practice in your hospital? Do you have a preference?

Episiotomy This is a cut performed under local anesthetic to enlarge the opening to the vagina and

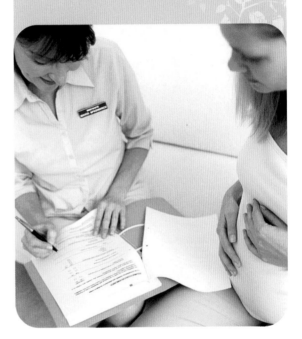

avoid natural tearing. If you are going to have a ventouse (vacuum extraction) or forceps delivery, it will be performed automatically.

Things to Think About: The Birth

Assisted delivery Despite your best efforts, you may need help to deliver your baby safely. The doctor can explain the advantages and disadvantages of the methods available in your hospital so that you can choose.

Position for delivery Make it clear in which position you'd like to deliver your baby (see page 138).

Things to Think About: After The Birth

Cutting the umbilical cord Would you or your partner like to cut the cord? You can also ask to see the placenta after the birth.

The way your baby is delivered Do you want your baby placed on your stomach or lifted into your arms as soon as s/he is born? Research suggests that initial skin-to-skin contact can be beneficial to the bonding process.

Cleaning and bathing of your baby Would you like the nurse or midwife to clean and dry your baby and wrap him or her in a blanket?

Vitamin K Some hospitals give newborn babies vitamin K in order to prevent a rare but serious blood

disorder, either by injection or by mouth. This is not compulsory.

Delivering the placenta Some hospitals offer a drug to separate the placenta from the womb after giving birth. If you do not want drugs, you must say so in advance so that a midwife who is experienced in "non-active management" of the third stage can be involved.

Feeding your baby Do you want your baby put to the breast right away?

The above information is only food for thought. You can include all or none of these points, and you can, of course, add your own specific preferences and requirements to the plan.

Prenatal Checkups

It is so exciting when you get a positive reading from a home pregnancy test kit and realize that you are expecting a baby. Once the initial euphoria has worn off, it is important to get your home-test results confirmed and to enter the health system that will monitor and help you throughout your pregnancy.

Your choice of prenatal and childbirth care will depend to some extent on what state you live in and the type of health insurance (if any) you have. Most women with private insurance will be under the care of an obstetrician and give birth in the hospital to which he or she is attached. But some women opt to be under the direct care of a nurse-midwife (part of a hospital obstetric team) or an independent midwife (this is usually for a home birth). Birth centers, run by midwives, are an option in some areas. Obstetrical clinics in teaching hospitals provide free or low-cost care for women who are willing to serve as "material" for medical students under the direction of specialists.

With this range of options, procedures during a pregnancy will naturally vary somewhat. Your own experience may differ from the following schedule, but it will probably be very similar.

Prenatal Schedule

As soon as you discover you are pregnant, make an appointment with your doctor or midwife. This first visit is usually scheduled for when you are at least eight weeks pregnant. At this time a pregnancy test will be done to confirm your results, and you may also be given a pelvic examination. At this and following appointments you may be given information about

- your baby's development during the pregnancy
- nutrition and diet
- folic acid and vitamin D supplements (see pages 58–59)
- lifestyle factors that could affect you and/or your baby, such as smoking, drinking, and recreational drug use (see pages 52 and 72)

- food hygiene
- exercise and Kegel (pelvic-floor) exercises
- your prenatal care
- prenatal classes
- prenatal screening tests (see page 96)
- planning your labor
- your options for where to have your baby

At the first appointment, you should discuss with the doctor or midwife any family history (on either your or your partner's side) of inherited diseases, such as cystic fibrosis; if anyone in your family has previously had a baby with an abnormality, such as spina bifida; or if you are being treated for a chronic condition, such as diabetes or high blood pressure. If this is not your first pregnancy, you should also point out if you had any complications or infections in a previous pregnancy or delivery.

During the early stages of your pregnancy, your doctor or midwife should

- give you your hand-held notes and plan of care
- identify any potential risks associated with your work
- measure your height and weight and calculate your body mass index

FIRST APPOINTMENT
Go to see your doctor as soon as you know that you are pregnant, in order to get all the necessary checks and tests during your first trimester and to ensure that you are given an appointment for your first ultrasound scan. Ideally, this visit should take place before 10 weeks.

- measure your blood pressure and test your urine for protein
- offer you screening tests, if applicable, and explain what's involved
- offer you an ultrasound scan at 8–14 weeks to estimate when your baby is due
- offer you an ultrasound scan at 18–20 weeks to check the physical development of your baby and screen for possible abnormalities
- take blood samples to check for blood group, hemoglobin levels (to check for anemia), and immunity to rubella (if you have no immunity, you will be offered a postnatal vaccination). Diabetes, hepatitis, syphilis, and your Rh status will also be tested

8–14 week ultrasound scan

Often known as a 12-week or dating scan, the main purpose of this scan is to work out how many weeks pregnant you are and to estimate your due date. The scan can also check that your baby has a heartbeat and is developing normally and if you're expecting twins, triplets, or more.

The scan takes about 5–10 minutes. The sonographer will put some gel on your tummy and will move a small hand-held device, called a transducer, over your skin to get views of your baby. Finally, you'll be given a report of the scan, which will tell you exactly how many weeks pregnant you are.

Some hospitals offer a nuchal translucency scan to all women at 11–14 weeks. A nuchal translucency test is used to assess the risk of Down's syndrome and other chromosomal disorders. Using ultrasound to check for abnormal thickness in the fold at the back of the baby's neck (nuchal), this test (when combined with a blood test) is 80–90 percent accurate in predicting Down's syndrome.

FETAL HEARTBEAT

When you hear your baby's heartbeat for the first time, it is such an emotional moment. Usually from about 16 weeks onward (sometimes earlier), your caregiver may be able to listen to your baby's heartbeat. However, it is no longer recommended as part of routine prenatal appointments. This is because it can be uncomfortable if your caregiver has to press into your bump to locate the heartbeat, and hearing the heartbeat doesn't tell you how healthy your baby is. However, if you want to hear your baby's heartbeat, your caregiver can provide this, if you ask.

Some midwives use an old-fashioned Pinnard stethoscope, which looks like a small horn, to listen. She'll hold one end to your tummy and the other to her ear. However, most obstetricians and midwives now use a hand-held Sonicaid fetal heart monitor, which amplifies your baby's heartbeat so you get to hear it, too. If you do get to hear the heartbeat, don't be surprised at the speed—your baby's heart rate is 120–160 beats per minute (BPM) compared to your 60–100.

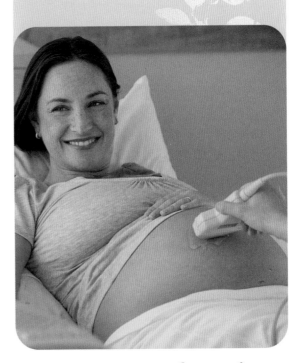

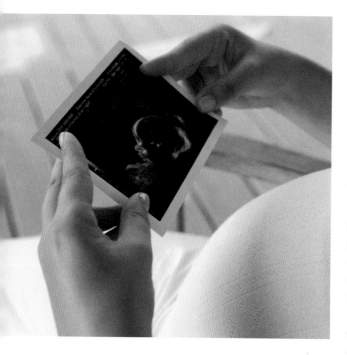

greenfile
Your blood pressure is lower in the middle of your pregnancy than at other times. It's perfectly normal, but if you get up quickly, you may find yourself feeling slightly light-headed as a result.

18–20 week ultrasound scan

You will be offered a detailed scan, known as the mid-pregnancy or anomaly scan, when you are between 18 and 20 weeks pregnant, to check that your baby is developing normally and to have a look at where the placenta is lying in your uterus. Measurements will be taken of your baby's head, spine, heart and other organs, hands, feet, arms, and legs.

Most hospitals allow you to watch the scan, which takes about 15 minutes, as it is being performed, and some allow you to buy a photograph of your unborn baby in the womb.

25 week checkup (first-time mothers only)

Your doctor or midwife will check the size of your uterus, measure your blood pressure, and test your urine for protein.

28 week checkup

Using a tape measure, your midwife will measure the size of your uterus. Your blood pressure and a urine test will be taken. If you are Rh-negative, your first anti-D treatment will be offered (see right).

31 week checkup (first-time mothers only)

The size of your uterus will be measured, your blood pressure taken, and a urine test for protein will be done. If you have had any screening tests since your last appointment, the results will be discussed.

34 week checkup

Your doctor or midwife should give you information about preparing for labor and birth, including how to recognize active labor, how to cope with pain in labor and your birth plan. S/he should also do

16 week checkup

Your doctor or midwife will talk to you about the ultrasound scan and any screening tests that you have had, measure your blood pressure, and test your urine for protein. If you are anemic, an iron supplement may be considered. You may also discuss the 18–20 week ultrasound and any concerns or questions you may have about it.

REGULAR CHECKS

Your urine and blood pressure will be checked at every prenatal appointment.

Urine is analyzed principally to check if protein, or "albumin," is present. If so, it may mean that you have an infection that needs treating. It can also be a sign of preeclampsia.

A blood pressure reading of 140/90 or above in pregnancy indicates high blood pressure. A rise in blood pressure later in your pregnancy (combined with protein in your urine) could be a sign of preeclampsia, a complication that can cause premature labor and stillbirth if left untreated.

the routine tests and measurements for the size of your uterus, blood pressure, and urine. If you are Rh-negative, you will then be offered a second anti-D treatment.

36 week checkup

You will receive the routine checks for size of uterus, blood pressure, and urine, and the position of the baby will also be checked. You may discuss what happens after your baby is born, including feeding and caring for your newborn, vitamin K and screening tests for your baby, your own health after the baby is born, and postpartum depression and "baby blues."

38 week checkup

The size of your uterus will be measured, your blood pressure taken, and your urine tested for protein. You might also discuss the options and choices available if your pregnancy lasts for more than 41 weeks.

40 week checkup (first-time mothers only)

This checkup is identical to the one you received at 38 weeks and is to reassure you and the medics that all is well.

41 week checkup

Naturally, no one wants to be at this checkup, but if you run over your due dates, it is at this appointment that you will discuss the options and choices for induction of labor. You may also be offered a membrane sweep, along with the routine tests and measurements for uterus size, blood pressure, and urine.

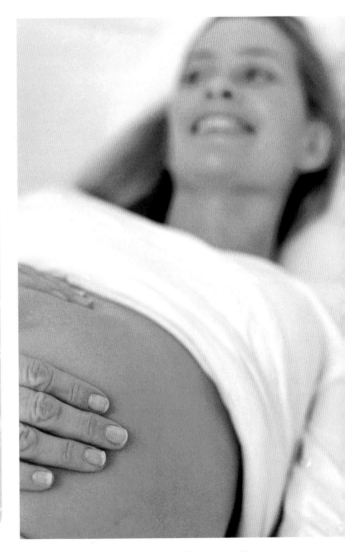

ANTI-D TREATMENT

Blood tests will show if you are Rh (rhesus) negative, but the medical team cannot know if your unborn child is Rh-positive or negative.

If your baby is Rh-positive and any of the baby's blood cells mix with yours, your body may start to produce antibodies against the rhesus D positive factor (antigen). This is not usually dangerous in first pregnancies. However, these antibodies can cross the placenta and attack the blood cells of the unborn baby, causing hemolytic disease of the newborn (HDN). This is generally a mild condition but it can be more serious and cause anemia or jaundice. Very rarely, it can cause stillbirth, severe disability, or death after birth.

Anti-D treatment during your pregnancy is offered as a precaution, and the implications and options available to you should be fully discussed so that you can make an informed decision about the treatment.

Prenatal Screening and Testing

All pregnant women are now routinely monitored throughout their pregnancy at prenatal visits, and tests that were once performed only if problems were suspected are now used more commonly. Some of the screening tests are more invasive than others.

A natural practitioner would recommend the use of basic tests, which are performed at a prenatal visit. This may include urine testing, checking blood pressure, measuring the growth of the uterus abdominally using a tape measure, and listening to the baby's heartbeat with a Pinnard stethoscope (see page 93).

However, those who favor a natural approach to prenatal care have reservations about the use of invasive—and they would say sometimes unreliable—procedures that have become routine in some places.

These prenatal screening tests to detect fetal abnormalities have their place and can prove extremely useful, depending on the circumstances. It can be an immense relief to find out your baby is growing well, for example; and screening can also provide lifesaving information when a problem is suspected.

However, it is also important that every woman know that prenatal testing is not obligatory and that she educate herself about the advantages and disadvantages of each test so that both she and her partner can make up their own minds about which tests they want done and which to refuse, if they deem it unnecessary.

Before making a decision about whether or not to undergo a test, it is also worth considering what you might do with the information if the test results were positive. You must weigh the risks and benefits of having these tests, especially if you plan to keep the baby no matter what the problem is. Support and counseling are available for all parents in these emotionally difficult situations (see Useful Contacts, page 156).

OLDER MOTHERS

In the developed world during the past few decades the average age of first-time mothers has been rising. For example, in the United States in 1970 it was 21.4 years of age, according to the National Center for Health Statistics, whereas in 2006 it was 25. In the same period the proportion of first births among women 35 and older rose from 1 in 100 to 1 in 12.

Unfortunately, the odds of having a baby with a genetic defect increase as you get older. Figures from the American Medical Association show that the risk of Down's syndrome in a baby born to a woman age 20 is about 1 in 1,667; at age 30 it is 1 in 952; at age 40, 1 in 106; at age 45, 1 in 30.

If you're almost, or over, 40, you should strongly consider genetic testing, such as chorionic villus sampling, amniocentesis (see right), or the quadruple tests, because the risk of genetic problems increases significantly. Your caregiver can give you full details of what these tests involve and the risks they may incur.

However, bear in mind also that many women who have delayed pregnancy until they're over 35 are surprised to find that, given generally good health, they're not much more likely than younger women to have serious complications, and the vast majority of women end up having healthy babies.

Chorionic Villus Sampling (CVS)

This procedure is used to detect chromosomal and genetic disorders, such as Down's syndrome and sickle-cell anemia. At 8–12 weeks, a tube is inserted through the abdomen or cervix and tissue is taken from the uterus and the tissue surrounding the embryo.
Advantages Accurate results within 48 hours.
Disadvantages Possible damage to the embryo, cervix, and uterus, with an approximate risk of miscarriage of 1 in 100.

Amniocentesis

Under local anesthetic, a long, sterile needle is inserted through your abdominal and uterine walls into the amniotic fluid, and a sample is taken. This test is conducted at 16–18 weeks to provide information about certain birth defects, such as Down's syndrome and cystic fibrosis. Results take about 2–3 weeks.
Advantages Extreme accuracy (c. 90 percent), and for gender-related disorders, it reveals the baby's sex.
Disadvantages Amniocentesis cannot screen for all defects, and it can cause miscarriage (less than 1 percent). It can also cause discomfort and side effects, such as bleeding and infection.

Alpha-Fetoprotein Test (AFP)

This blood test checks blood protein levels and can detect neurological problems, such as spina bifida and hydrocephalus.
Advantages Noninvasive with no side effects.
Disadvantages Although not harmful, this test has a high rate of false positives and is only 50 percent accurate. You are then frequently referred for further screening—probably an amniocentesis—with a higher risk factor.

---

greenfile

The optimum time to perform an AFP test is between 15 and 18 weeks, when the test is thought to be most accurate.

ULTRASOUND SCANNING

The vast majority of American women have at least one scan during pregnancy and probably two, but it is not compulsory. If you'd rather not have a scan, you should discuss this with your caregiver; and the final decision rests with you. However, it is worth bearing in mind that ultrasound scans give reliable and useful information about your pregnancy, and many women find it reassuring to see their baby moving on screen.

There has been a growth in the number of clinics that offer obstetric scans, and both 3D and 4D ultrasound scan technology is now widely available.

The 3D ultrasound produces a lifelike picture of your baby built up from images of the three "planes" of vision as stored in the computer after the ultrasound. A 4D ultrasound is a moving or "video-style" image of your baby in the womb.

Apart from the financial considerations (check your health insurance), there is no restraint on how many private scans an expectant mother can undergo. However, although there is no medical evidence that ultrasound scanning can harm an unborn child, some believe that more long-term research is needed.

Due to this lack of research, some experts suggest that the ultrasound scanning is more appropriately reserved for essential, diagnostic use only—for example, to investigate a suspected placenta previa (when the placenta is lying unusually low in the uterus), to assess a baby with a significant size/dates discrepancy, to determine fetal position if palpation cannot establish this, or to check that the fetus is still alive, if this is a question.

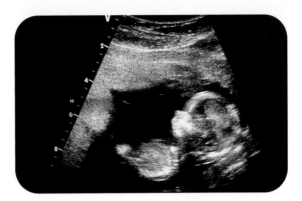

Natural Birth Education Classes

Prenatal classes, or childbirth classes, as they are also known, are a very good way to prepare yourself for your baby's birth and to meet other pregnant women who are due around the same time as you and who are based in your local area.

There is a wide choice of prenatal classes available to you—more, of course, if you live in a large town or city. You may find one at your local hospital, or your doctor or midwife may be able to recommend a class. It's a good idea, if you're considering a particular class, to ask a woman who has attended it if she found it helpful. The quality of the teaching may be more important than the approach advocated by the class.

First-time mothers, in particular, enjoy the opportunity of talking to other women, as well as professionals, about their worries and concerns. Talking with others in the same situation can be a real help. Depending on the topic being discussed that week, partners are also welcome at some classes, and this can be illuminating for both of you, because you may find you can talk more openly in a group discussion.

Naturally, the information and support you gain from these classes can help you to make informed decisions about the kind of labor and birth you might like to have. However, another significant benefit is that prenatal classes are a wonderful way to make friends with local women in similar situations and at the same stage in life that you have reached—and you'd be surprised how much, and how often, these friendships can help you through the first few months of living with a new baby. Some can last a lifetime.

Choosing a Prenatal Class

You should have some intuitive idea of what you would like to gain from a prenatal class so that you can choose the kind of class that best suits your needs—such as a class that embraces natural birth options and pain relief, or one that concentrates more on a conventional approach.

LAMAZE

Lamaze promotes a natural, healthy, and safe approach to pregnancy, childbirth, and early parenting.

Lamaze antenatal classes help to break down and simplify the birth process while providing key information you need to know to have a safe, healthy birth. Lamaze education is designed to help you work effectively with your healthcare provider so that together you can make decisions that are right for you, and ensure a safe and healthy childbirth experience.

For further details and to find a class near you, check out their website (see Useful Contacts, page 156).

Start looking for a class quite early in your pregnancy, since places may get booked up well in advance. You can, of course, choose more than one class, if you want a broader take on your options. Talk to your midwife, health visitor, or doctor about what is available.

Many childbirth classes also cover breast-feeding and early baby care.

What to Expect

Classes are typically held once a week and last for about one and a half to two hours, either during the day or in the evening. The atmosphere is generally relaxed and informal.

Some classes are open to women only. Other courses welcome all parents and parents-to-be, including young parents, women without a partner, same-sex couples, and surrogacy couples. Women who are not attending with a partner are sometimes welcome to bring someone else along to classes—for example, a friend or family member.

Most women start attending about 8–10 weeks before their baby is due. Bear in mind that if you're expecting twins (or more), you might like to start the classes earlier, since you'll probably deliver before your due date.

The range of topics usually covered in prenatal classes includes

• health in pregnancy
• suitable exercises during labor
• what happens during labor and birth
• coping with labor and different types of pain relief
• self-help techniques for labor and birth
• relaxation techniques
• how to give birth without intervention, if that's what you want
• information on different kinds of birth and intervention
• emotional changes in pregnancy, and the early postnatal period
• your health after the birth
• caring for your new baby, including feeding

Not all classes are able to cover all of the above topics—some choose to concentrate on certain aspects, so it's worth checking course content before registering.

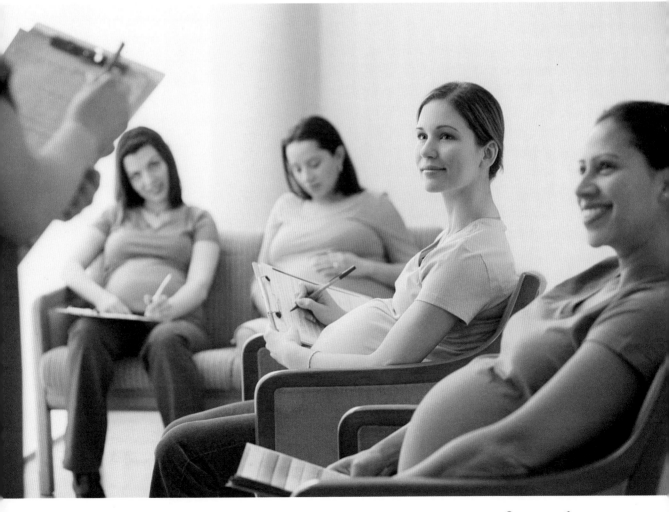

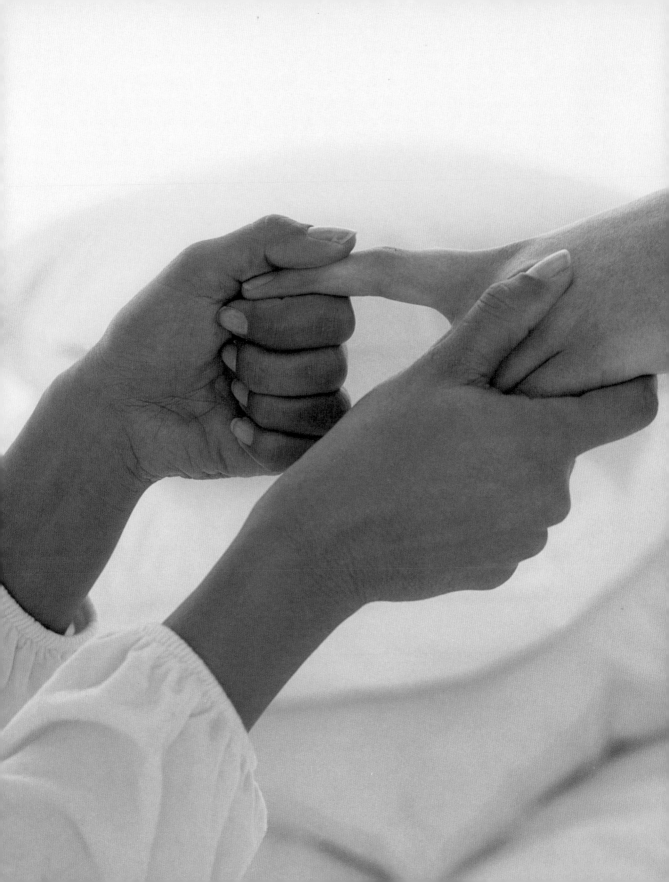

6

Remedies
& Therapies

There are numerous complementary therapies and natural treatments available that can help to relieve many of the common ailments of pregnancy, helping you to enjoy the optimum mental and physical health possible.

Complementary therapies can help you prepare for the birth, provide pain relief in labor, ease nursing difficulties, and help you through the early days of parenthood. Yet it brings peace of mind to know that an obstetrician or pediatrician is available should the need arise. An integrated approach, combining conventional prenatal care provision with complementary therapies, can often bring the best and most pleasing results.

In this chapter, we seek to give you a basic overview of some of the complementary practices that are most appropriate during pregnancy, so that you can confidently choose the therapy that is right for you.

The therapies range from manipulative treatments that involve a hands-on approach, such as reflexology and osteopathy, through energy therapies, such as reiki and use of flower essences, to medicinal therapies that involve taking drops, tinctures, or teas, such as homeopathy and herbalism.

Each therapy has its own governing body, and it is essential that you check the credentials of any practitioner—make sure that they have the right qualifications and insurance, and follow the code of ethics. For further details on a particular therapy or for a list of local practitioners, contact the relevant individual association (see Useful Contacts, page 156).

Chiropractic

Chiropractic treatment involves manipulating the body's joints, with emphasis on the spine, in order to relieve irritation on the nerves that run through the center of the spinal column. Considered an alternative medicine, since its development at the end of the nineteenth century, its benefits are now more widely recognized by medical practitioners. Chiropractors believe that if a vertebra is displaced, it may press against nerves and so cause an imbalance, resulting in discomfort, pain, or even disease.

greenfile

Chiropractors who routinely treat pregnant women usually have a chiropractic table with a breakaway pelvic/abdominal section. When your bump becomes too big for you to lie face down comfortably, this allows your belly, and consequently the baby, to remain unrestricted during the adjustment. After the fourth to fifth month, you should never lie on your stomach for an adjustment without this type of table, or without the use of a pregnancy cushion or pillow.

BENEFITS OF CHIROPRACTIC

Pregnancy: Chiropractors can help relieve spinal or back problems caused by physical and chemical changes in a woman's body when she is pregnant. Treatment can also relieve symptoms of nausea, sciatica, and lower back and pelvic pain, especially in late pregnancy. A chiropractor may also offer advice on how to adapt your lifestyle in order to make daily routines easier.

Postnatal mothers: Treatment is recommended for back problems associated with a difficult birth, reduced sleep, and lifting the new baby. Childbirth can also cause your upper back musculature to become tight, interfering with proper nerve flow to the breasts. By chiropractic adjustment of the spine following delivery, milk can flow properly, decreasing breast-feeding problems.

Chiropractic treatment is drug free and uses gentle pressure and manipulation of the spine to relieve painful conditions. Realigning the spine during pregnancy releases uterine nerves so that they can function properly. Treatment is carried out by means of precise adjustments, in a way similar to osteopathy (see opposite). There are many similarities between the two therapies, but a slight difference lies in the emphasis placed on soft tissue and spinal manipulation techniques. Chiropractors are also trained to take and read X-rays.

What to Expect at a Consultation

After taking details of your medical history, a chiropractor will ask you to adopt various positions in order to evaluate your spinal function. He will use gentle manipulation to correct any misalignment and may use a gentle thrust to free a joint.

Chiropractors are able to give tips on proper back exercises and nutrition to help you have a comfortable and healthy pregnancy. Depending on your condition, you can expect to attend for up to six sessions, or for routine visits each month. A chiropractor who is versed in the needs of pregnant women will also provide you with exercises and stretches that are safe to use during pregnancy and will complement any adjustments made to your spine.

Osteopathy

Osteopathy uses manipulative techniques and massage to restore and maintain the musculoskeletal system (the bones, joints, muscles, ligaments, and connective tissue), easing muscle tension and restoring joint mobility and balance. Since your changing shape and increasing weight affect this balance, osteopathy may be of real benefit in relieving the aches and pains of pregnancy.

There are several specializations within osteopathy, including cranial osteopathy, which uses very small movements and manipulation of the head. These work with the anatomy and physiology of the patient to effect changes and to allow health to be restored.

What to Expect at a Consultation

After taking a full medical history and reviewing your lifestyle and your emotional health, an osteopath will check your posture, mobility, and weight distribution. He will then form a diagnosis and treatment plan, which may include manipulation and massage.

An osteopath can monitor your changing body throughout your pregnancy, making adjustments as necessary, with a final appointment six weeks after the birth of your baby.

Treatment may consist of massage, manipulation, stretching, and, occasionally, what is known as the "high velocity thrust"—a vigorous technique used to free up a joint, although this is not commonly used during pregnancy. Treatment is not usually painful, although it can feel a little uncomfortable.

> According to a recent survey, more than 80 percent of moms-to-be experience back pain at some time during their pregnancy.

BENEFITS OF OSTEOPATHY

Pregnancy: With its emphasis on maintaining the musculoskeletal system, osteopathy is most often used to relieve backache during pregnancy, but it is also helpful for correcting "pregnancy posture" and treating morning sickness, piles, swollen legs and hands, and for moving the baby into a more comfortable position. In the latter stages of pregnancy, osteopathy can help sciatica, pubic pain, ligament pain, restricted mobility, swollen ankles (edema), and carpal tunnel syndrome.

Postnatal mothers: Osteopathy is used to help both mother and baby recover after the shock of the birth, and treatment is sometimes available in the hospital in the days following delivery. In the few months after giving birth, problems such as stress incontinence or shoulder pain from breast-feeding can also benefit from osteopathic treatment.

WARNING Although osteopathy is safe throughout pregnancy, many osteopaths avoid giving treatment at the transition from the first to the second trimester (about 12 weeks), because this is a vulnerable time.

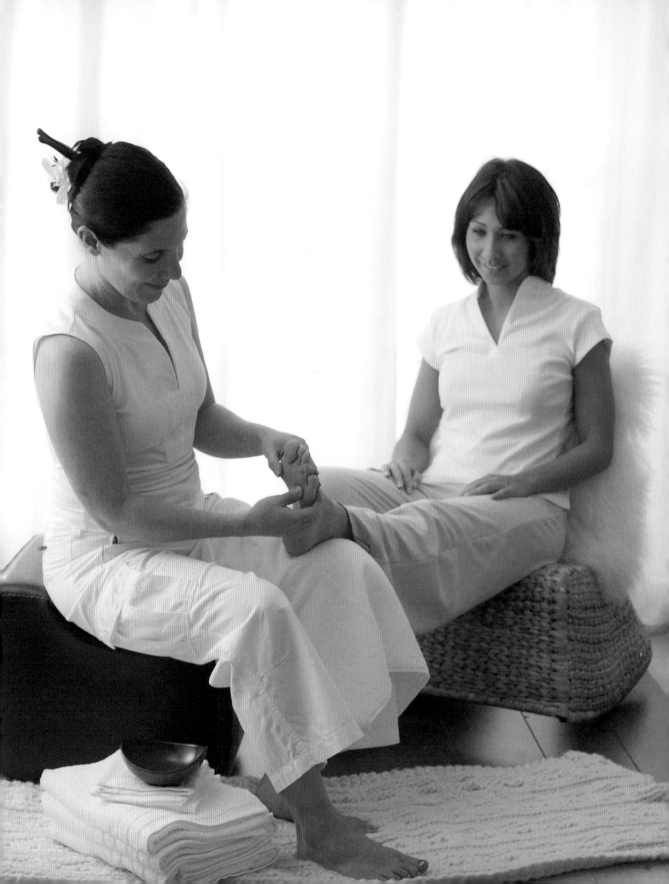

Reflexology

Loosely based on ancient eastern foot massage therapies, western reflexology involves the gentle manipulation of the feet (or occasionally hands) to stimulate the body's own healing process.

The underlying principle is similar to that of acupuncture (see page 108) in that each pressure point on the sole or sides of the foot correlates with a particular function or part of the body. However, the meridians or zones of the body are described differently in reflexology from the way they are described in acupuncture. In reflexology, every organ and system of the body has a corresponding "reflex point."

Reflexologists believe that applying pressure to specific points on the foot stimulates the corresponding part of the body to get rid of toxins, allowing the body to heal itself.

Reflexology is suitable for a wide range of pregnancy conditions but is particularly appropriate for any circulation or stress-related problems and for pain management.

What to Expect at a Consultation

Although reflexology is not a diagnostic tool, it does look at the underlying causes for symptoms, so your initial treatment will probably address you as a whole, rather than purely your specific ailment.

Reflexology is a noninvasive therapy, and you will merely be asked to take off your shoes and socks. The treatment should be relaxing, as the therapist exerts a firm pressure with the thumb on each reflex point, working from toe toward ankle. However, you may experience some pricking pain occasionally or a bruised sensation as an area that correlates to an affected organ or region is worked on.

Some people experience a slight reaction to treatment the following day—perhaps mild flulike symptoms or a slight skin rash. This is a sign that the body is beginning to detoxify and heal itself, and the reactions should pass fairly quickly. Another common side effect is more frequent urination after a treatment—something you know all about when you're pregnant anyway. Weekly sessions are recommended—usually for about six weeks, depending on the condition. Each session lasts about an hour.

greenfile

Reflexology can work extremely well alongside orthodox treatment for common pregnancy ailments.

BENEFITS OF REFLEXOLOGY

Pregnancy: Reflexology has a good track record for treating conditions such as stress, backache, morning sickness, headache, constipation, cystitis, and raised blood pressure.

Labor: Great for pain control when giving birth and to reduce the length of labor.

Postnatal mothers: Again, good for control of chronic pain and dealing with the discomforts and minor conditions associated with the period just after giving birth.

WARNING Reflexology is not suitable if you have a history of miscarriage or if there's a risk of fetal loss, preeclampsia, or placental disturbance. Care should be taken in the first trimester of pregnancy, and you must tell your practitioner that you are pregnant. You should consult a qualified practitioner before attempting any self-help techniques.

Aromatherapy

Aromatherapy uses essential plant oils to improve physical, mental, and emotional health and to prevent disease. The oils can be administered by massage, inhalation, compressions, and/or baths.

Essential oils can be very potent, and not all are safe to use during your pregnancy (see below). It is therefore important to find a qualified aromatherapy practitioner who can recommend particular oils to treat your condition and give indications of the doses to be used. You can choose to benefit from aromatherapy by inhaling the oils or via an aromatherapy massage (see page 38).

What to Expect at a Consultation

After a discussion about your medical and lifestyle history, an aromatherapy practitioner will select oils for their specific effects and may blend as many as five oils together for optimum results. These oils are then diluted in a carrier oil, such as sweet almond oil, before being applied to your skin, usually in the form of a therapeutic massage.

Note that the following oils should be avoided during pregnancy: aniseed, arnica, basil, clary sage, cypress, fennel, jasmine, juniper, marjoram, and rosemary.

BENEFITS OF AROMATHERAPY

Pregnancy: Oils can be used to ease symptoms such as lower back pain and to give temporary relief from sciatica. They are also beneficial for stress relief and relaxation. When working in conjunction with doctors and midwives, aromatherapy can be used to help edema, or swelling.

Labor: Some oils can assist with the labor and have an effect on the uterus and uterine muscles. For instance, jasmine helps the uterine muscles and also gives confidence. If you don't want to be massaged, you can always burn oils in the delivery room to good effect. If a burner is not permitted, oils will vaporize well in hot water in a small room.

Postnatal mothers: If you have stitches, a few drops of lavender oil in the bath are very beneficial, due to its natural healing and antiseptic qualities. Geranium also helps with hormone balance. These oils must be used in a very low dilution while you are breast-feeding.

Many pregnant women have successfully used aromatherapy on themselves during their pregnancy to alleviate common ailments, but caution must be exercised. You should always use the best quality organic oils you can buy and follow instructions carefully. Consult your doctor or midwife before using essential oils.

greenfile

Mothers report that regular aromatherapy massage during pregnancy results in babies who are calm and good sleepers.

WARNING Some essential oils should not be used for the first 14–16 weeks of pregnancy, and some remain contraindicated throughout the full term (see above). A qualified aromatherapy practitioner can give details of dilutions for massage, but these are generally very low during pregnancy (about 5 drops of essential oil to 4 tablespoons of carrier oil), and for infants. Expert advice should always be sought and followed.

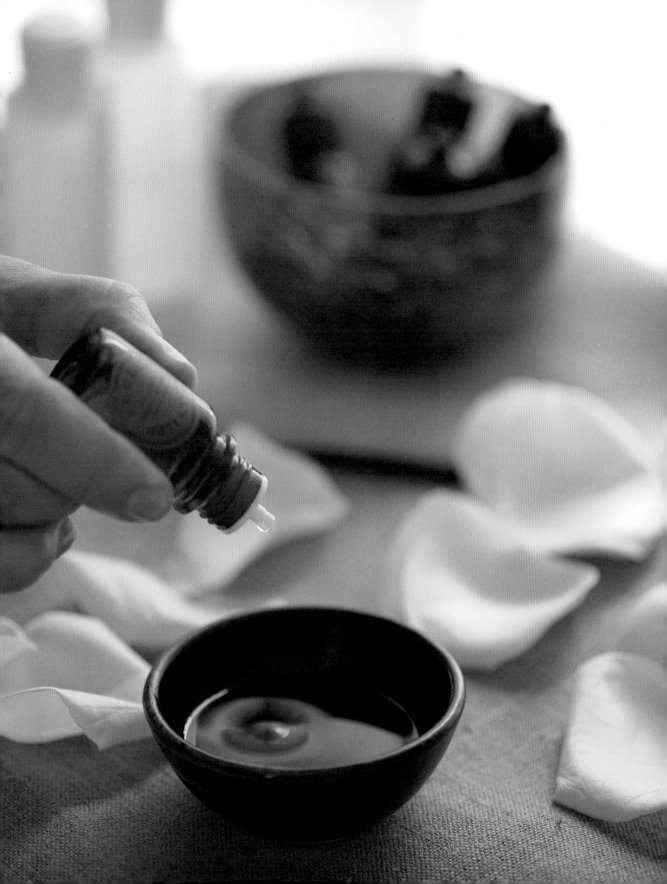

Acupuncture

One of the best known and respected of complementary therapies, acupuncture is, in fact, part of the comprehensive system of traditional Chinese medicine (TCM), which dates back thousands of years. However, in the West, acupuncture is often used in isolation, and many conventional health professionals have learned the techniques.

The philosophy behind TCM and acupuncture is completely different from western medical thinking. According to Chinese belief, the key to health lies in the balance of two opposing forces (yin and yang, the passive and active forces). Achieving balance and harmony is the fundamental objective of this complex and sophisticated system of medicine. It emphasizes the close interaction of mind and body.

Healthy balance relies on the smooth flow of vital energy known as qi (pronounced "chee") through channels, or meridians, in the body. Imbalance or ill health occurs when there are blockages or weaknesses in the flow of this energy, or if outside influences, such as excessive heat, cold, or damp, get into the body.

Acupuncture involves using very fine needles, inserted at strategic points (acupoints) on the body to stimulate the flow of vital energy and to correct imbalances. There are other noninvasive alternatives (see right).

What to Expect at a Consultation

Treatment is preceded by very careful questioning and observation. The practitioner will look at how you move, your complexion, body shape, and so on. S/he will listen carefully not only to the answers to his questions but to how you answer—your tone and how you respond. The practitioner will closely inspect your tongue and will also feel the six pulses on your wrists (three on each, according to TCM) and will take down details of your medical history, lifestyle, sleep patterns, eating habits, likes, and dislikes.

From this, he will decide on a course of treatment, often using a combination of acupuncture, herbs, and

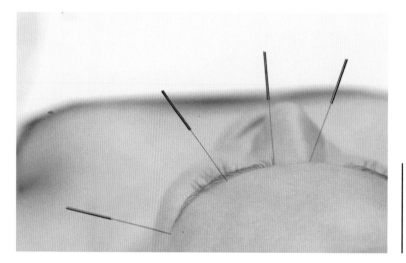

WARNING Make sure you inform your practitioner that you are pregnant before treatment commences, as certain acupoints should not be stimulated during pregnancy.

occasionally moxibustion (in which herbs are burned over an acupoint without touching the skin). You generally require between six to ten treatments before you see improvement in your condition.

Although it is natural to worry about whether having needles stuck in you may hurt, actually all you should feel is a pinprick as the needles are inserted and perhaps a slight sensation of tingling or numbness. Initially, the needles are left in for 6–10 minutes, building up to 20 or 25 minutes in later sessions. Don't be surprised if you feel somewhat sleepy after a session; this is entirely normal.

greenfile

The name "moxibustion" is derived from the Chinese word for mugwort, moxa, which is the herb that is dried and burned in the treatment.

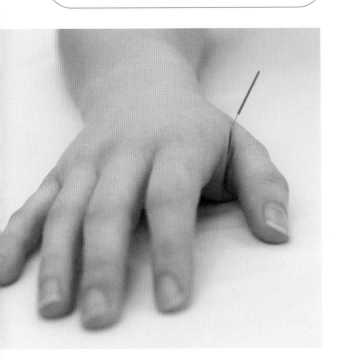

BENEFITS OF ACUPUNCTURE OR ACUPRESSURE

Pregnancy: Either treatment can help relieve common pregnancy problems, such as morning sickness, nausea, constipation, hemorrhoids, varicose veins, heartburn, and backache, and are also effective against many conditions that you may have had prior to pregnancy for which you can no longer take medication, such as stress-related problems or migraine.

Labor: Often used when breech presentations need turning and for those who have gone over term and don't want to be induced. Treatment starts around week 41 and during the days between then and going into hospital for an induction. Sometimes an acupuncturist will go into the hospital once the waters have broken to try to get the labor going.

However, acupuncture and/or acupressure are used during labor mainly for pain relief and can have a significant effect—ideal if you want a totally natural birth. Acupuncture can also be used to help the placenta deliver naturally without the need for an injection.

Postnatal mothers: Acupuncture is very successful in the treatment of hemorrhoids. It is also useful to help you get your strength back and to treat physical problems, such as mastitis, as well as emotional problems, such as "baby blues" or even postpartum depression.

ACUPRESSURE

If you are concerned by the idea of having needles inserted into you, acupressure is an effective alternative; in this technique the therapist applies gentle pressure to the acupoints in place of needles.

In recent years, laser or ultrasound acupuncture has also become more popular, since with these new techniques, nothing actually breaks the skin.

Reiki

Reiki is a form of healing therapy that was devised in Japan in the early twentieth century by Dr. Mikao Usui, after years of research and meditation. It is used primarily for stress reduction and relaxation and to promote healing.

Reiki practitioners are trained to channel reiki healing energy through their hands to wherever it is needed in the patient's body. They achieve this by laying their hands on or over specific areas of your body.

The treatment is able to address physical, mental, emotional, and spiritual problems and to stimulate your body's own healing powers to restore balance. Reiki practitioners believe that the body absorbs the help that it needs and that the healing energy travels directly to the source of the problems, giving relief from symptoms, deep relaxation, and mental and emotional harmony.

What to Expect at a Consultation

A treatment usually lasts about an hour. The practitioner will ask you to lie with your eyes closed on a raised couch (you remain fully clothed) or occasionally to sit on an upright chair. The practitioner then holds her hands on or just above your body, moving them to various positions where her hands may remain for some time before moving on.

BENEFITS OF REIKI

Pregnancy: Reiki is helpful in easing back pain, sciatica, and headaches and for dealing with emotional conditions, such as anxiety and stress. It is also said to be good for preparing the body and mind for the birth.

Postnatal mothers: Reiki is believed to help relieve emotional "blockages" and to help you to deal with any negative thoughts.

---

greenfile

Reiki has grown in popularity at a remarkable rate in recent years, and there are many newly qualified practitioners with limited experience. Make sure you consult a reiki master who is well practiced and who knows that you are pregnant (see Useful Contacts, page 156).

WARNING Currently in the U.S. there is no formal accreditation of reiki training based on approved national standards. Some medical centers do include reiki practitioners, and you might check with your local hospital to see if it does. Otherwise, your best option is to rely on personal recommendation.

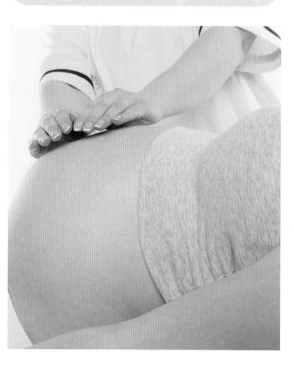

Hypnotherapy

Hypnosis works with your subconscious mind to help overcome unwanted habits of physical responses. Your conscious mind can focus on only one or two things at once, whereas your subconscious is much bigger and is constantly processing information and storing it.

Hypnotherapy is growing in popularity for pregnant women because it is completely noninvasive, it has no side effects, and it can be used safely when other options are limited.

If you have an emotional concern, such as a fear of childbirth or a needle phobia, you could benefit from hypnotherapy. In addition, hypnotherapy can help with physical problems, such as heartburn, water retention, and nicotine or alcohol dependency. For help during labor, hypnobirthing is now a recognized option (see page 148).

Self-hypnosis techniques can be taught to you by a hypnotherapist, which can be useful for deep relaxation and relieving stress.

What to Expect at a Consultation

The practitioner will talk to you about your health and any problems you may be encountering. You will then be put into a hypnotic state, where you will feel deeply relaxed while your practitioner talks to you in a slow, soothing voice. It's likely that you will be fully aware of everything going on around you, but you will feel at ease. Contrary to popular belief, a hypnotherapist cannot make you do anything you don't want to do, and you can stop the session at any time.

greenfile
Under hypnosis, you can visualize your baby, rather like a 3D scan but in your own mind.

WARNING Always consult a fully qualified, registered hypnotherapist (see Useful Contacts, page 156).

BENEFITS OF HYPNOTHERAPY

Pregnancy: Excellent results with discomfort, high blood pressure, heartburn, water retention, stress and anxiety, fear of the birth, needle phobias, and addictions, such as helping you to give up smoking or alcohol.

Labor: Useful for turning breech babies, for natural induction, and for preparing for a cesarean section.

Postnatal mothers: Helpful for rapid healing after birth, postpartum depression, and bonding with your baby.

Studies in the United States and Australia show that hypnosis can help with relaxation, postpartum depression, and managing discomfort. Some hospitals in Australia have begun working with hypnotherapists in prenatal support.

Research published in the *British Medical Journal* showed that nicotine in patches can still cross the placenta; however, hypnosis is a completely safe way of trying to quit smoking.

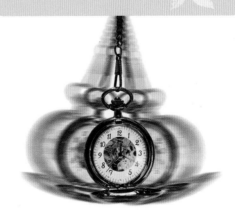

Medical Herbalism

During your pregnancy, you may be drawn to herbalism as a nontoxic alternative to conventional medicines. In fact, herbs have been used for thousands of years to ease pregnancy symptoms and the pain of labor.

Modern scientific interest in herbalism stems from a growing awareness that synthetic drugs may have unpleasant, and sometimes serious, side effects. Many doctors accept the validity of herbalism, and some herbalists work alongside conventional physicians (although they are not licensed to practice medicine in the United States). Meanwhile, research is being carried out into the plant-based folk medicines of the native peoples of South America, Africa, China, Siberia, and elsewhere.

Today, scientists find, extract, and then synthesize in the laboratory a single active constituent from a plant—the part that has therapeutic value. That ingredient is then manufactured on a large scale for use in pharmaceutical drugs. Herbal drugs, however, are extracts from sections of the whole plant, such as leaves, roots, and berries, and contain hundreds, perhaps thousands, of plant constituents.

Herbalists believe that the active constituents are balanced within the plant and are made more (or less) powerful by the numerous other substances present. For example, synthetic diuretics seriously reduce the potassium levels in the body, and this is restored using potassium supplements. The herbalist uses dandelion leaves, which are potent diuretics but also contain potassium to replace naturally that which is lost.

Each culture has its herbal tradition, but Chinese herbal medicine is now proving to be very popular in the West, particularly for the treatment of skin problems. Traditional Chinese medicine works with about 10,000 different herbs, often used in conjunction with acupuncture (see page 108). Western herbalists follow the same principles, using different, indigenous plants.

While Chinese herbs are especially popular for treatment of skin problems, practitioners can treat

BENEFITS OF MEDICAL HERBALISM

Pregnancy: Many of the usual complaints that crop up during pregnancy, such as morning sickness, constipation, headaches, tiredness, skin problems, and hemorrhoids, will respond to herbal treatment, when prescribed by a professional.

Labor: Increasingly women are using herbs in the form of herb teas, tinctures, or essential oils to facilitate a smooth labor. If you want to use herbs during labor to influence contractions (hypertonic or stalled, for example), you should consult a practitioner. A professional, who can reliably liaise with other health professionals if necessary, will then be on hand throughout your care.

Postnatal mothers: You can use herbs after the birth of your baby for physical and emotional support. There are herbs to aid recovery from the impact of giving birth, to help wound healing, to strengthen the system when the demands of breast-feeding hit you, and to soothe frazzled nerves when it all feels too much!

Useful herbs to enhance milk flow in breast-feeding mothers are raspberry, fennel, and nettle. Herbs for lifting the spirits include lemon balm, lavender, and Saint-John's-wort. However, significant, prolonged postpartum depression needs to be treated by a qualified practitioner.

WARNING Although some plant-based treatments for minor ailments—particularly herb teas or infusions—are widely available and are generally regarded as harmless, other plant derivatives are potentially dangerous and should be administered only under the guidance of a professional medical herbalist. Certain plants and herbs should be avoided during pregnancy, and anyone with liver disease, such as hepatitis, or high blood pressure should consult a doctor before taking Chinese herbs.

all physical conditions that don't require surgery or manipulation, and psychological problems as well. Many conditions are treated with a combination of herbs and acupuncture; the acupuncture relieves immediate symptoms, while the longer term herbal treatment will restore the balance of the body.

What to Expect at a Consultation

In Chinese medicine, the diagnosis will be made from looking at your tongue, taking the pulses in the wrists, and observing your general appearance. Western medical herbalists are trained in the same diagnostic skills as orthodox doctors but take a more holistic approach to illness. The underlying cause of the problem is sought, and, once identified, it is this that is treated rather than the symptoms alone.

Herbal treatments may be prescribed in the form of a tincture (an alcohol-based liquid), a cream or compress, or a dried herb powder from which to make a tea. This should be taken several times a day as prescribed. Treatment may include advice about diet and lifestyle as well as the herbal medicine.

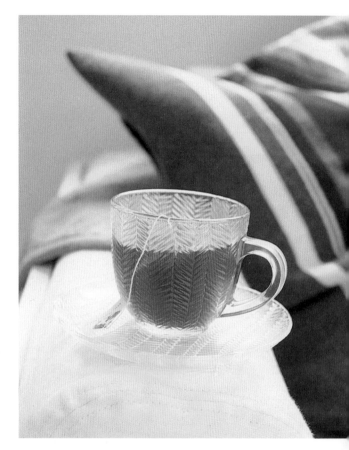

HERBAL SELF-HELP

There are certain gentle tea infusions that may be taken in moderation throughout pregnancy. For example, you can sip ginger tea, made from fresh gingerroot steeped in hot water, to quell the nausea of morning sickness. Similarly, chamomile tea for relaxation is safe throughout. However, as a general rule, take herbal or plant remedies only under professional supervision.

On the other hand, herbal compresses and poultices are completely safe, yet very beneficial, because they are applied topically. For example, a cold witch hazel or nettle tea compress applied directly to hemorrhoids brings immediate relief.

Some women swear that taking raspberry leaf (*Rubus idaeus*) as a herbal tea can bring on labor and make it easier, and even that it can help to restore the uterus to its nonpregnant state after the birth.

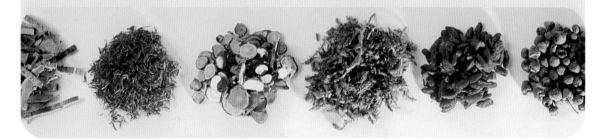

Homeopathy

As a nontoxic alternative to conventional pharmaceutical drugs, homeopathy is, not surprisingly, a popular choice of treatment for pregnant women. Homeopathy was founded by a German doctor, Samuel Hahnemann, in 1796. It is based on the belief that "like may cure like"—a theory similar to that underlying vaccination or immunization, in which the body's natural resistance is stimulated by a remedy that mimics the symptoms.

The basis of homeopathic treatment is to stimulate the body's own healing processes to cure the particular ailment or overpower the bacteria, rather than treating the symptoms themselves.

Homeopaths emphasize that they treat people, rather than diseases, and that a human being is more than the sum of his/her physical parts. Homeopathic medicine is said to be suitable for both acute and chronic conditions.

A minute amount of the active ingredient is used in a specially prepared form, which means homeopathic remedies cannot cause side effects and you cannot become addicted to them. Many of the remedies are produced from herbs or plants, although conventional drugs can also be prescribed homeopathically—that is, in very small amounts. Homeopaths believe that the more dilute the concentration, the more powerful and effective it is.

What to Expect at a Consultation

Your homeopath will start by taking a detailed case study, including your past medical history and finding out about your general energy levels. An initial consultation may last an hour or more. Your homeopath will then prescribe a homeopathic remedy, usually in tablet or powder form for adults, or as a liquid remedy for infants. Further appointments last about half an hour.

During treatment, you may experience a period of exceptional well-being and optimism. Alternatively, you may develop a cold, rash, or some form of discharge, which means your system is going through a cleansing stage. Sometimes symptoms can appear to get worse for a short time—don't be alarmed as this is usually a sign that the remedy is taking effect, but always check with the homeopathic practitioner that this is a normal reaction.

greenfile

Certain substances, such as coffee, eucalyptus, menthol, spearmint, and peppermint (including many proprietary toothpastes and mouthwashes, so use natural products), can neutralize homeopathic remedies and should be avoided.

The designation 6c or 30c after the name of a remedy refers to the amount of dilution. So, a 6c potency can be repeated more frequently.

WARNING Although over-the-counter remedies are available, you should never self-prescribe homeopathic treatment. In all cases, it is recommended that you contact a qualified homeopath for advice and treatment (see Useful Contacts, page 156).

In fact, if you have any response to the treatment that concerns you, contact your homeopath right away. You may also want to make notes of any changes and take them with you to discuss at your next appointment.

The number of consultations required depends very much on the individual. Generally, acute conditions respond more quickly, and the longer a chronic illness has existed, the longer it will take to disappear.

FINDING A HOMEOPATH

Although homeopathy is less widely accepted in the United States than it is in some other countries, such as Britain, there are many qualified practitioners in this country. Some specialize in homeopathy, while others also hold degrees in other branches of medicine. Your health insurance may cover homeopathic treatment. A good starting point, if you wish to find a homeopathic doctor, is to go to the web site of the National Center for Homeopathy (see Useful Contacts, page 156).

BENEFITS OF HOMEOPATHY

Pregnancy: There are remedies to treat minor health problems associated with pregnancy, such as mild urinary problems, diarrhea, anemia, varicose veins, backache, and thrush, or emotional upset, and to help alleviate nausea and sickness, tiredness, cramps, and heartburn. Homeopathy can be used to turn a breech baby and to ensure that the labor and birth go smoothly by dealing with anxiety and fear, and also to tone the uterus.

Labor: Suitable remedies can help produce strong effective contractions, stimulate the uterus if it fails, and deal with exhaustion and irritability.

Postnatal mothers: Homeopathic remedies can aid a fast recovery from damage to delicate tissues and from exhaustion and bruising. Homeopathy can also help establish a good flow of milk for breast-feeding mothers and help protect the nipples from cracking and soreness. It is also excellent for treating mastitis. There are specific remedies to help with baby blues and anxiety.

If you are given homeopathic remedies to take at a later date, be sure to store them in a cool, dark place, away from anything with a strong smell. If you travel, do not let the remedies go through the X-ray machines at airports.

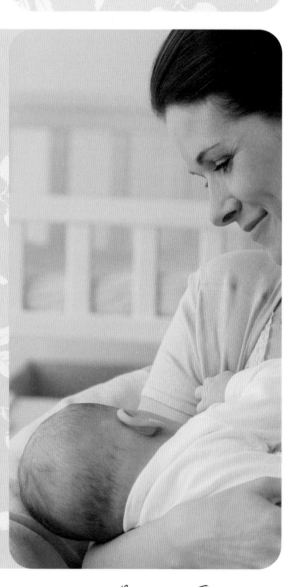

Shiatsu

Also known as Japanese "finger pressure" therapy, shiatsu originates from the same oriental principles as acupuncture (see page 108) combined with a western knowledge of physiology.

Like acupressure, shiatsu works by manually stimulating the body's vital energy flow (known as "ki" in Japanese) in order to promote good health. However, in shiatsu, the practitioner uses thumbs and fingers, elbows, and even knees and feet to apply pressure and stretching to the energy lines known as meridians.

Physically, this has the effect of stimulating the circulation and the flow of lymphatic fluid, working on both divisions of the autonomic nervous system, helping to release toxins and deep-seated tension from the muscles and stimulating the hormone system. On a subtler level, shiatsu allows you to relax deeply and get in touch with your body's healing abilities.

What to Expect at a Consultation

A personal case history will be recorded before the treatment. The *hara* is a very important diagnostic tool for shiatsu. For this, the practitioner will gently probe your abdomen to map the energetic state of your body, its organs, and the corresponding meridians.

A shiatsu treatment is normally given on a padded mat at floor level or on a futon, while you lie, fully clothed, either prone, supine, or on your side. You may also receive part of your treatment sitting in a chair or on the mat. The massage should be pleasurable and relaxing, not uncomfortable.

The practitioner may give advice on diet, exercise, and lifestyle, encouraging self-understanding and greater independence in health matters. Your shiatsu practitioner may also offer you a personal health assessment. This will be an insight into your condition but does not constitute a medical diagnosis as such.

greenfile

You will get more from your treatment if you avoid eating a large meal, taking strenuous exercise, or having a hot bath or shower just before or after a shiatsu treatment.

After shiatsu, you will probably feel invigorated yet relaxed. While patients generally experience increased well-being, there may be temporary healing reactions as toxins and negative emotions are released; these may take the form of a headache or flulike symptoms for 24 hours. In such cases, contact your therapist.

Most practitioners recommend more than one shiatsu treatment to secure lasting improvement to health problems. A session lasts about 45 minutes.

BENEFITS OF SHIATSU

Pregnancy: Good for relieving morning sickness, vomiting, and constipation, shiatsu is also commonly used to relieve headaches, neck and shoulder pain, back pain, sciatica, cramps, digestive problems, stress, fatigue, and depression. In later pregnancy, it can help alleviate edema, or swelling.

Labor: Can help to trigger labor if you are overdue, and can help to control pain.

Postnatal mothers: Helps with postnatal aches and pains, back and shoulder ache from breast-feeding, and other common complaints.

WARNING Make sure your shiatsu practitioner has experience of working with pregnant women and knows to avoid certain acupoints during pregnancy. Always choose a qualified practitioner (see Useful Contacts, page 156).

Flower Remedies

It was as recently as the 1930s that German homeopath Edward Bach revived the ancient therapeutic use of flower remedies as first recorded by the ancient Egyptians. Perhaps his best-known variety is the flower blend known as the Bach Rescue Remedy, which is often used for shock or panic, but which is also very good for calming the mind as the birth approaches.

Since the 1980s and the renaissance of complementary therapies, flower essences have grown in popularity, and now native plants from around the world, such as the Australian Bush remedies, are readily available in stores worldwide.

The therapeutic properties of the plants are harnessed by infusing them in spring water and preserving their essence in alcohol. Flower essences can be used to treat your emotional and spiritual state, but also physical conditions, as symptoms of ill-health are often considered a manifestation of problems on a higher or emotional level.

What to Expect at a Consultation

Flower remedy practitioners tend to work in their own specific ways. Many are intuitive healers who use dowsing to find the right combination of flower essences for you. Other practitioners rely on hearing a detailed account of your emotional and mental state and personality before prescribing a combination of essences to help you to deal with your situation.

Your practitioner may make up a bespoke remedy containing the prescribed essences for you, or you may be advised to buy the relevant individual essences. Both the made-up prescribed remedy and the individual essences are then diluted in mineral water or fruit juice, to be taken several times a day until the condition improves.

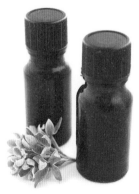

BENEFITS OF FLOWER ESSENCES

Pregnancy: Ideal for helping relieve emotional states, such as stress and anxiety, sleeplessness, depression, or fear, and physical complaints, such as pain or shock.

Labor: Rescue Remedy is often used to calm the mind and ease pain and shock.

Postnatal mothers: Flower essences are excellent for helping you deal with the spectrum of emotions that new mothers experience, ranging from exhaustion to feelings of overwhelming responsibility.

FLOWER ESSENCES FOR PREGNANCY AND BIRTH

Walnut, for adjustment to change

Watermelon and zucchini, for a harmonious pregnancy

Mimulus, for fear of pain or things going wrong

Rockrose, for terrifying thoughts

Forget-me-not and Pineapple weed, for bonding with your baby

Star of Bethlehem, for shock after a traumatic birth

WARNING Flower essences are safe to take through all stages of pregnancy, but since most are preserved in alcohol, it's important to follow dosage instructions carefully and not to exceed recommendations.

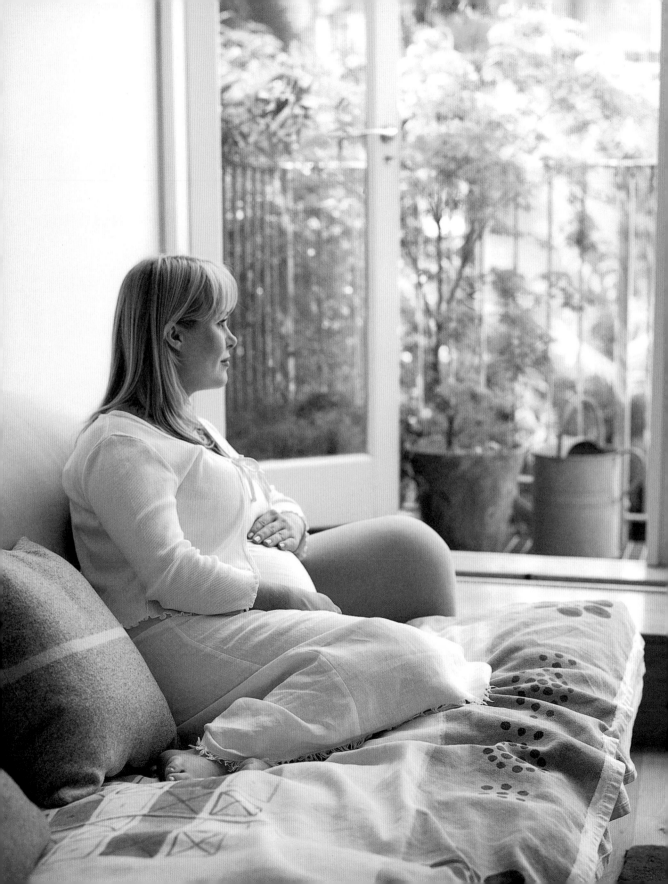

7 Health & Well-being

Pregnancy is the time in your life when you are forced to review your approach to health and healing. Given that many of the conventional medicines are no longer available to you, it is the perfect time to think about using a natural remedy to alleviate your health problems. This chapter looks at the common complaints you may experience during pregnancy and offers suggestions on ways to treat and relieve them naturally. You are still vulnerable to everyday illnesses, such as coughs and colds, and without recourse to conventional medicines it's good to know that there are some alternatives available. With the rush of hormones that accompanies pregnancy and the anxieties that may come and go, you may feel particularly vulnerable to your emotions, and there are therapies and remedies that can help you experience a positive pregnancy.

Natural medicine is gentle and effective. It will work with your body to deal with illness in the way that nature intended, without causing any harm to your unborn baby. No one is suggesting that you turn your back on conventional medicine. It has a valuable role to play in your prenatal care, but very often you can successfully help and heal common ailments using tried-and-tested natural medicines without resorting to your doctor. This integrated approach to illness offers the best of all worlds.

NOTE The advice in this chapter should not be considered as a substitute for medical advice from your family doctor or any other qualified medical practitioner. If you treat yourself with natural medicines, such as herbs, you should always inform your doctor, because these can be very powerful and interact with prescribed or over-the-counter medications.

Common Pregnancy Complaints

There are a number of minor yet discomforting complaints that are common during pregnancy. You may be lucky and escape them, but it's probably worth stocking up on a couple of basic natural ingredients that will help you to tackle the unpleasant side effects of conditions such as morning sickness, fatigue, and cramps efficiently yet naturally.

Morning Sickness

Just over half of all pregnant women complain of morning sickness at some point in their pregnancy, most commonly during the first three months. Symptoms are often experienced on awakening in the morning, although morning sickness can strike at any time of the day or evening. Symptoms include nausea, vomiting, excessive salivation, and a disinclination to eat.

Although morning sickness is unpleasant but mild for most women, some can be more seriously affected, becoming dehydrated and vitamin-deficient from excessive vomiting.

There is no definitive answer to what causes morning sickness and why some women get it while others don't. Theories include hormonal fluctuations, emotional reactions to pregnancy, nutritional factors and biological mechanisms that cause your body to reject substances that may cause the baby harm. Some believe that it's the body's way of eliminating toxins and that, as a result, those who suffer from morning sickness actually have a healthier pregnancy.

HOMEMADE GINGER TEA
Grate a 1-in (2.5-cm) length of peeled, fresh gingerroot into a mug and pour freshly boiled water over it. Leave to infuse for 5 minutes. Strain, add a squeeze of lemon and honey to taste, and sip slowly when cooled. Drink two or three times throughout the day to relieve symptoms.

What to do

The first course of action should be to avoid smells and foods that nauseate you (often spicy, gas-producing, or fatty foods). Choose foods that appeal to you and regularly eat small, nutritious snacks, while drinking plenty of water to keep yourself hydrated.

Sipping herbal teas can offer relief from morning sickness. Ginger tea is the most common remedy (see above), but other herbal teas, such as chamomile, fennel, spearmint, or peppermint, can be soothing and are able to relieve sickness.

Complementary therapies enjoy good results in the treatment of morning sickness (see page 100).

acupressure self-help
When feeling nauseous, press strongly with your thumb on the Pericardium 6 acupoint, which is located on the inside of your forearm at a point two thumb widths above the crease of the wrist and between the tendons.

greenfile
Keep a snack by your bed overnight, so that you have something to eat before getting up in the morning. In my experience, a couple of ginger cookies first thing did the trick.

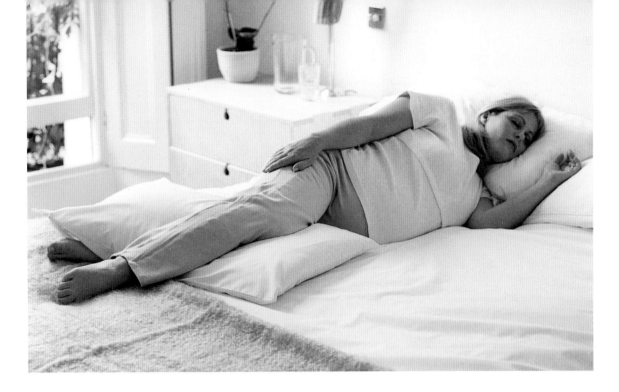

Fatigue

Given the fact that your body is working overtime to help develop a new life inside, it's small wonder that you suddenly feel as if you have no energy. This is normal, and you shouldn't be alarmed at all.

There are some sensible precautions you can take to help reduce the impact of this sudden fatigue, and some recommendations that may help you to sail through the acclimatization period while you adjust to the changes in your body and psyche.

What to do

To increase your energy levels, try boosting your diet with iron-rich foods, together with foods high in vitamin C to help increase absorption (see page 44). Drinking nettle tea two or three times a day is another good way of boosting iron levels.

Make sure you are getting plenty of sleep. If you still feel tired, take a nap. Learn to listen to your body and rest when you need to without worrying about the "things that need doing."

Conversely, taking a brisk walk in the fresh air is also an excellent way of increasing your oxygen intake and improving your circulation, so combating fatigue. In fact, any moderate exercise, inside or outside, can be invigorating and help to banish fatigue.

Don't be tempted to raise energy levels by snacking on energy-rich, sugary foods, such as chocolate, or stimulants, such as coffee; this is a quick-fix, which will offer only temporary respite! By the same token, even herbal stimulants should be avoided during pregnancy. A better choice is to get some proper rest or nourishment and consider concentrated food supplements, such as spirulina and molasses (see page 59).

greenfile

A few drops of lemon, orange, or sandalwood essential oil added to your morning bath can be invigorating and refreshing to both mind and spirit.

WARNING If you feel consistently exhausted and irritable, this could be an indication that you are anemic. Consult your doctor or midwife for advice.

Heartburn

More than three-quarters of pregnant women suffer at some point from heartburn, a burning sensation in your chest and throat. Hormonal changes can soften the valve between the esophagus and the stomach, allowing food and gastric juices to return into the esophagus with the accompanying burning sensation or acute pain in the chest.

The situation is compounded as the pregnancy progresses and the growing baby puts pressure on the stomach, making symptoms worse in late pregnancy.

Heartburn often occurs after meals or as a result of eating the wrong food, but it can be alleviated by sensible eating and gentle, soothing herbs.

What to do

Try eating frequent, smaller, low-fat meals to reduce the symptoms of heartburn. You should favor alkaline foods, such as fruits and vegetables, over acidic foods (see right) and try to avoid spicy, greasy, and sugary food. Some experts believe that a combination diet—for example, eating proteins and carbohydrates separately and at different times of the day—can help to relieve heartburn.

It is also recommended that you eat a light evening meal early in the evening, say around 6 p.m., and have a small snack before going to bed, if required, rather than eating a large meal late in the evening.

Complementary therapies, such as acupuncture, reflexology, homeopathy, aromatherapy, and herbalism, all report good results in the treatment of heartburn (see pages 100–117).

Sometimes lying down can aggravate heartburn, so sleep with one or more pillows under your head.

ALKALINE AND ACIDIC FOODS

Most raw fruit and vegetables are alkalizing foods, with the exceptions of cranberries, pomegranates, strawberries, plums, corn, broccoli, and asparagus. Apple cider vinegar is alkalizing, while distilled white vinegar is acidifying. Almonds and chestnuts, and seeds, such as pumpkin, sunflower and flax, are considered to be alkaline foods. All herbal seasonings are considered to be alkalizing.

Nearly all cooking oils and all grains are considered to be acidifying foods, as are coffee and chocolate. Cheeses made from cow's, goat's and sheep's milk are acidifying foods, as is butter. Most animal sources of foods, including tuna, shrimp, salmon, and cottage cheese, are considered to be acid foods. All alcoholic beverages make the acid food list, as do any forms of pasta.

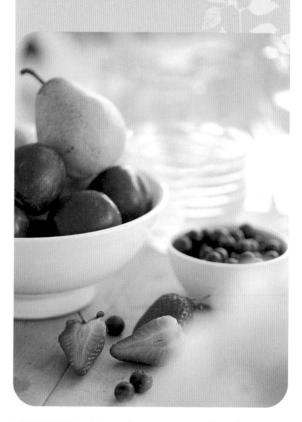

greenfile

Slippery elm or dandelion tea is an excellent way to relieve the pain of heartburn. You can also take slippery elm lozenges.

WARNING Avoid over-the-counter antacids and medicines, and even baking soda, which are contra-indicated during pregnancy.

Leg Cramps

Mildly painful leg cramps, often at night, are common during the second and third trimesters. They usually occur as a result of the extra weight that you are carrying, a lack of exercise, or a calcium or magnesium deficiency.

Not all women experience leg cramps but, rather, have an uncomfortable, achy, restless, or pulling sensation in their legs. These are simply milder symptoms of the same condition.

What to do

You can very easily reduce the frequency of leg cramps by taking a few simple remedial steps.

Firstly, try to build more activity into your daily routine and, at the same time, improve your mineral intake, either by eating more calcium and magnesium in your diet (see pages 45 and 48) or by taking supplements. Vitamin E is also said to reduce cramping.

Often you can relieve a leg cramp by massaging and stretching your leg muscles. Flex and point your foot as you massage to release the tension.

Soak your feet and calves, if possible, in a warm footbath to which you have added a few drops of arnica.

greenfile

Lack of salt in your diet can cause muscle cramps, so although it is not normally necessary to salt your food, if you suffer from cramps, try sprinkling a little sea salt on your dinner.

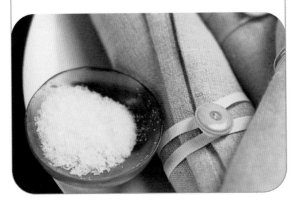

Seventy-five percent of pregnant women get stretch marks.

Skin Problems

Some women report that their skin improves thanks to the hormonal changes of pregnancy, but others are affected by itching and other skin troubles.

If you are eating a healthy, balanced diet, you may well avoid or reduce the discomfort of some of the more common skin problems. However, there are measures that you can take to alleviate many skin conditions.

What to do

Itchiness You may experience intense itchiness as the skin of your belly, breasts, and thighs stretches. In addition, the liver is working harder to process the increased hormonal load, and this can cause the skin to itch. Make sure your skin is well cleansed with mild natural soap or simply with clean, warm water. You can exfoliate with a loofah or soft body brush to stimulate circulation and leave the skin soft and clean. Moisturize well, using cocoa butter or vitamin E lotion. To reduce itching, use calendula oil or apply echinacea tincture mixed half-and-half with water.

CHLOASMA

Also known as the mask of pregnancy, chloasma is a darkening of the skin predominantly on the forehead, nose, and cheeks below the eyes. This is not dangerous but can cause embarrassment for some women. Aloe vera gel is said to help lighten these areas during pregnancy, but the darkened patches should return to their normal color after childbirth.

WARNING After 28 weeks, if you experience severe, persistent itchy skin, consult your doctor, as this could be an indication of obstetric cholestasis, a rare but serious condition that must be treated with conventional medicine.

Stretch marks These cannot necessarily be prevented, but a diet rich in zinc, found in ginger, cheese, and whole grains, for example, is said to help. If the telltale silvery lines start to appear, you can nourish the area so they become less pronounced using vitamin E, almond or wheatgerm oil, or herbal oils containing chamomile, mandarin, calendula, or rose.

Sore Breasts

Even before you have confirmed that you are pregnant, you may experience tender, sore, or tingly breasts with extremely sensitive nipples. This acute sensitivity usually subsides by the end of the first trimester, but many women report that their breasts feel heavy and tender throughout the pregnancy due to their increased size. It is important to wear a supportive bra throughout your pregnancy (see page 80).

What to do

Soaking in a warm bath with the water covering your breasts can offer temporary relief from discomfort and heaviness. You can alleviate tenderness in early pregnancy by massaging your breasts once or twice a day with a soothing herbal oil. Try mixing several drops of rose geranium or arnica essential oils into a base oil of sweet almond (3 oz [90ml]) for a soothing massage oil.

Swelling

Mild swelling, or edema, particularly of the feet and ankles, is quite normal during pregnancy, especially toward the latter stages. Hot weather, prolonged standing, or fatigue can all aggravate the situation.

Normal swelling should reduce after you rest and in the morning when you wake up.

What to do

Preventive measures are best when dealing with edema. Make sure you raise your feet when sitting for about 20 minutes, three or four times a day. If possible, periodically lie down with your feet above your heart level to help circulation. Similarly, you should avoid standing for extended periods, especially in hot weather.

Regular exercise enhances circulation and helps to avoid or reduce swelling.

When sleeping, try to lie on your left side to improve circulatory function.

Constipation

Virtually all women, especially those who are overweight, experience constipation during pregnancy, because the hormone progesterone slows bowel movements. To add insult to injury, the combination of constipation together with increased rectal pressure due to the weight of the baby puts you at risk of hemorrhoids.

As with most ailments, prevention is better than cure, so a few adjustments to your daily routine may help you to avoid this uncomfortable condition, which is the root cause of so many other pregnancy complaints, including indigestion, headaches, and skin problems.

What to do

The most common cure for constipation is to use laxatives. However, you should avoid over-the-counter

WARNING The medical term for swelling is edema. However, if after you press your finger onto your legs or hands, you leave an indentation mark, this is called pitting edema, which may indicate a more serious condition. You should seek advice from your doctor in this case.

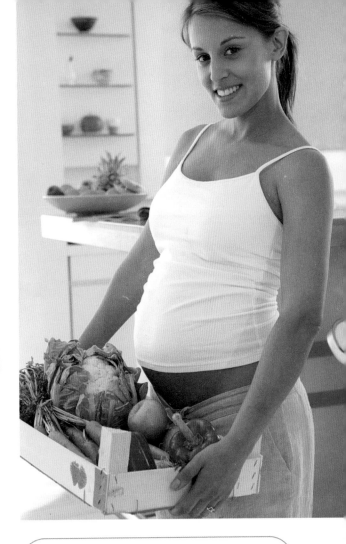

CONSTIPATION: PREVENTIVE MEASURES

Increase your physical activity—exercise helps to stimulate the muscle contractions in the colon.

Drink lots of water.

Drink a cup of hot water with a dash of lemon before breakfast.

Limit processed foods and caffeinated beverages.

Eat beets and cabbage—these are gentle laxatives.

Eat lots of fresh fruit and vegetables (at least some raw).

Give yourself time each day to sit on the toilet, relax, and wait.

Do not ignore your body's signal to empty your bowels—go to the toilet without delay.

To alleviate the pain of hemorrhoids, a traditional cure is to put grated potato or carrot directly on the affected area.

laxatives in favor of a mild natural laxative (although milk of magnesia is safe during pregnancy).

The most effective natural laxative that is safe during pregnancy is dandelion root tincture, which is available from health food stores and natural pharmacies.

A popular Ayurvedic (traditional Indian medicine) remedy for constipation is to drink a mug of hot milk mixed with a teaspoon of ghee (clarified butter) at bedtime.

You can also massage your abdomen to help stimulate bowel movement. You should recline on a bed, sofa, or even in a warm bath. Massage your abdomen quite deeply in a circular, clockwise direction, for about ten minutes. Then proceed to the toilet.

Some complementary therapies, such as acupuncture, homeopathy, herbalism, and nutritional therapy, are successful in the treatment of constipation and hemorrhoids (see pages 100–117).

WARNING Herbal laxatives such as castor oil, senna, buckthorn, and aloes should be avoided during pregnancy.

greenfile

Physiologically speaking, squatting is the best position for bowel movements. Strange as it may seem, actually squatting on the toilet seat—while exercising extreme caution—or sitting with your feet raised on a stool, or even on tiptoe, can assist the process.

For some women, eating bran (an excellent remedy for constipation, in fact) can irritate the intestine lining. Oats are a less harsh alternative, especially when cooked with raisins, so why not have a bowl of oatmeal to start the day?

Everyday Ailments

Before your pregnancy, everyday aches and pains or the symptoms of coughs and colds could be dealt with by the contents of your medicine cabinet. During your pregnancy, these conventional medicines or painkillers may be unsuitable, and you will need to find natural alternatives to ensure that you and your baby maintain a healthy, drug-free pregnancy.

Back Pain

Many pregnant women get backache, for numerous reasons, but if you suffered with back problems before your pregnancy, it is even more likely that you will get bouts of backache at this time.

The weight of your growing baby places a great deal of stress on your lower back muscles, and this can then be compounded by poor posture. In addition, urinary tract infections (see page 128) and constipation (see page 124) are common during pregnancy, and these can, in turn, lead to backache.

What to do

Any of the postural body work therapies, such as Alexander technique, yoga, qigong, and polarity therapy, are useful to correct your posture if backache is persistent.

If you can't attend a class, try to improve your posture yourself; avoid the habit of swaying your back to accommodate the weight at the front. Instead, stand up straight, tuck your tailbone under so that your pelvis is not tilting forward, and let your shoulder blades drop down your back. Try to correct yourself

greenfile

You can make an effective, warming poultice by mixing two cups of white breadcrumbs with a tablespoon of cayenne pepper and enough warm water to make a dough like consistency.

Position this on the affected area of your lower back, but do not leave on for more than 15–20 minutes, as the cayenne may burn the skin.

to this posture whenever you catch yourself slipping back into bad habits. (There is actually a medical term for the swayed back, belly-out position adopted by many pregnant women—it's called lordosis.)

Osteopathy and chiropractic are the best-known complementary therapies for back pain, but shiatsu and acupuncture are also recognized as being highly beneficial at bringing relief from the pain and discomfort of backache and sciatica (see pages 100–117).

Massage is also very helpful (see page 38). Obviously, a professional massage can help, but even if your partner or friend simply rubs your back using a little warm, gentle massage oil, this can help to give respite from the discomfort.

Remember to rest and take the weight off your feet (and pelvis) as often as you can with your feet up. Applying heat to the affected area (wrap a hot water bottle in a towel or use a wheat bag) can sometimes help. Following the same principle, soaking in a hot bath is also recommended.

SCIATICA

"Sciatica" is the medical term for a pain that travels from the lower back down the back of the leg, through the calf, and to the outer side of the foot. It is caused by inflammation of the sciatic nerve and is common in women in the later months of pregnancy.

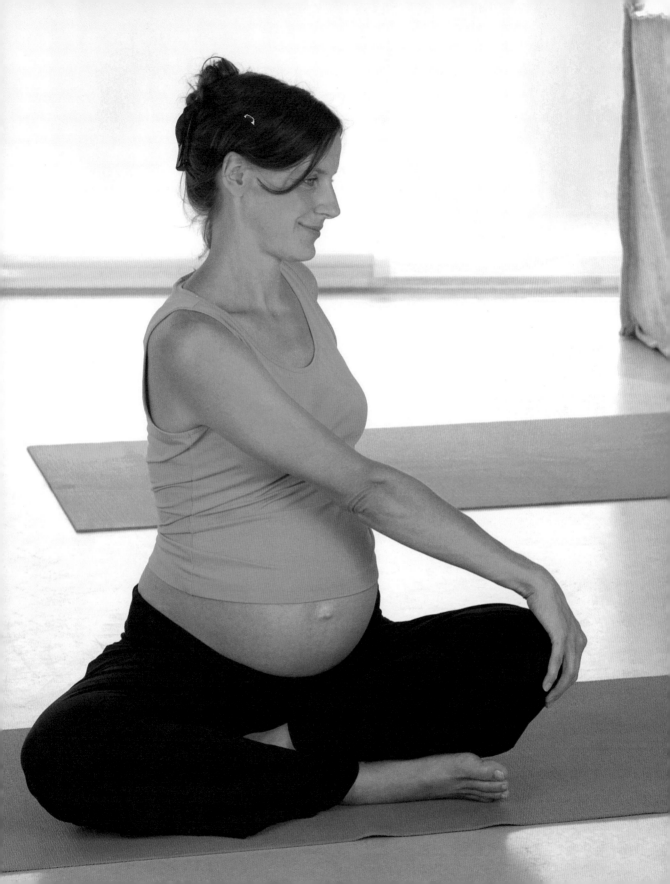

Colds and Flu

Although a common cold or influenza can be extremely debilitating during pregnancy, it should not be a threat to you or your baby. However, if you have a prolonged fever or high fever, you should consult your doctor. Otherwise, it's a case of making sure you get plenty of rest, eating highly nutritious and natural foods, and waiting it out while you treat the symptoms with natural cures.

On a cautionary note, if you have used herbs to treat a cold or flu when you were not pregnant, you may have to review your usual treatments, since some herbs are not safe for use during pregnancy. These are the ones also used in some aromatherapy oils (see page 38).

What to do

It is important that you remember to drink lots of fluids when you have a cold or flu, even if you don't really feel like it. If you become dehydrated, your kidneys will become overtaxed and your baby could be adversely affected. So, as a rule of thumb, you need to drink a cup of water, diluted fruit juice, or herbal or fruit tea at least every two hours—more if you're feverish.

NATURAL COLD REMEDY

A German friend gave me this recipe when I was pregnant with my first child, and I've used it for the relief of colds and sore throats ever since.

½ onion, sliced

2 cloves of garlic, chopped

½-in (1.5-cm) piece of gingerroot, chopped or grated

1 tablespoon olive oil

Sugar or honey, to taste

In a small pan, sauté the onion, garlic, and ginger together in the oil. Cover with cold water and bring to the boil. Reduce to a simmer and then add sugar or honey to sweeten. Strain and sip when cooled.

At the first signs of a cold, many women swear by the use of echinacea root tincture to reduce the symptoms and to limit the duration of the cold. There have been some concerns raised about the safety of echinacea during pregnancy; but to date, the evidence suggests that there is no increased risk of birth defects or other pregnancy-related health problems.

Sipping herbal or fruit teas can be effective for reducing the fever, aches, and discomfort of a common cold or flu. Try lemon balm, chamomile, or elderflower and, in moderation, ginger or dried yarrow. However, do not take yarrow during the first trimester.

Garlic is a natural bactericide and therefore useful in the treatment of many common ailments, including colds and sore throats. Taken in conjunction with vitamin C, it is particularly potent.

Cystitis

Also known as urinary tract infections (UTIs), cystitis is a common complaint that can affect you at any time, but it is particularly widespread during pregnancy, because the weight of the womb upon the bladder and ureters increases the likelihood of stasis (a stagnation in the normal flow), which breeds bacteria and can lead to infection.

Symptoms include frequent urination (sometimes hard to distinguish from the greater frequency brought on by pregnancy), often accompanied by burning sensation or pain on passing water. In some cases,

WARNING You should avoid sexual intercourse if you have cystitis.

you may also experience flulike symptoms, tenderness above the pubic bone, and, very rarely, vaginal bleeding.

Cystitis responds well to natural treatments, but if left untreated, it can become much more serious and develop into a kidney infection. This can be a serious threat to your health, and immediate attention from your doctor is required.

What to do

To ease cystitis, you should listen to the old wives' tale and drink cranberry juice. It has now been scientifically proven that cranberries prevent pathogenic bacteria from adhering to the wall of the bladder. If you can't get hold of fresh cranberries to make your own juice or smoothies, the best alterantive is to buy organic, pure cranberry juice (which you may have to sweeten) rather than the artificially sweetened commercial brands.

Besides cranberry juice, you should drink as much water as possible during the day to help flush the system.

If urinating is extremely painful, pour warm water over the entrance to the urethra as you sit on the toilet. Alternatively, urinate in a shallow bath (making sure to clean the bathtub well afterward). A warm bath with a couple of drops of chamomile, geranium, or lavender essential oil may ease cystitis symptoms.

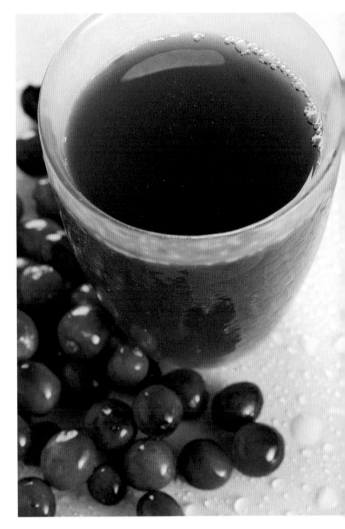

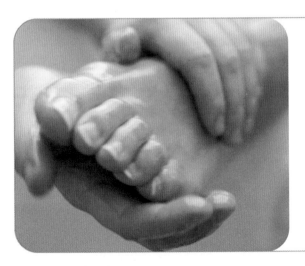

greenfile

Avoid eating beets, tomatoes, and citrus fruits when suffering from cystitis, as these are likely to aggravate the condition.

A reflexologist (see page 105) can stimulate the kidney, bladder, and urinary tract reflex points on the foot to try to disperse the toxins that are causing cystitis, so it may be worthwhile consulting one if the cystitis returns.

Headache

Normally, when you get a headache, you may take a couple of pain killers and continue with your day as usual. However, when you're pregnant, you cannot take your normal pain relief medication. During pregnancy, when you get a headache—and 10 percent of pregnant women suffer from more severe headaches or migraine—you have to rely on natural remedies, which can be just as effective.

What to do

Firstly, you should try to identify what is causing your headache. Is it linked to the hormonal changes that occur in pregnancy? Is it perhaps caused by stress or tension in the muscles of the head and neck due to poor posture? Is it a migraine, triggered by something you may have eaten or done?

Sometimes, getting some fresh air and taking a little exercise at the same time—perhaps a walk in the park, for example—is enough to lift a headache or to stop it developing.

Again, as with many of these everyday ailments, making sure you're getting enough sleep and rest is essential. Try to reduce stress levels if you think tension is the root cause of your headaches. You might like to try the meditation and relaxation techniques outlined on pages 36–9, as they are particularly good at relaxing tight muscles and relieving tension.

Some traditional midwives recommend taking a brief hot shower followed immediately by a quick blast of cold shower to relieve a headache, but it's not for the fainthearted. Often, a headache can be relieved by stimulating certain acupoints on the face and head. Try

> **SELF-MASSAGE TO RELIEVE**
> **MIGRAINE HEADACHES**
>
> Place the fingers of both hands on either side of the midline of the back of your neck, just under the base of the skull.
>
> With elbows raised and fingers perpendicular to the neck's midline, apply pressure to your neck muscles with your fingertips.
>
> Sweep up the neck, deeply massaging the neck muscles, and then back down the neck, massaging as you go.

using your thumb to apply gentle pressure to the point between your eyebrows, just above the bridge of your nose. You can also massage the part of the head that is hurting, using a gentle circular movement. You or a partner can extend the massage down the neck and shoulders to ease muscle tension and improve blood circulation.

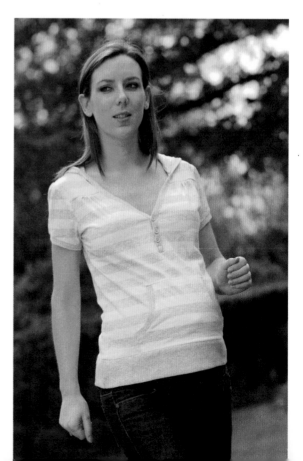

> ### greenfile
>
> Headaches are commonly caused in pregnancy by dehydration or low blood sugar levels. Drink plenty of water and keep a healthful snack with you.
>
> Try putting 3–4 drops of lavender oil on a compress and applying to the temples to relieve a headache.

Sore or Bleeding Gums

Changes in estrogen and progesterone levels can cause your gums to become inflamed, resulting in their bleeding when you brush or floss your teeth. In severe cases you can develop gingivitis, which often worsens as your pregnancy progresses. You should consult your doctor or dentist if you suspect you have gingivitis, since, if left untreated, it can cause serious gum and bone problems.

What to do

You can soothe sore or bleeding gums, which are common in the first half of pregnancy, by sipping chamomile tea or by rinsing the mouth with a chamomile infusion (see right).

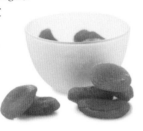

A diet rich in vitamin C can help to prevent gum problems. Good vitamin C food choices include apricots, citrus fruits, apples, cherries, watercress, brussels sprouts, and alfalfa.

In addition, the homeopathic remedies Kreosotum 6c and Phosphorus 6c are said to be effective for the relief of inflamed, swollen, or bleeding gums—seek advice from a trained homeopath (see page 114).

Carpal Tunnel Syndrome

This condition is caused by swelling in the hands, which restricts nerves in the wrist. It is particularly common in the third trimester. You may experience numb, tingling or painful fingers, often worse at night.

What to do

Acupuncture, shiatsu, homeopathy, and osteopathy (see pages 108, 116, 114, 103) are all useful therapies for treating carpal tunnel syndrome, and a physiotherapist can provide splints to support the wrists. However, you can also follow some self-help techniques to ease this painful condition. Try gently circling and flexing the wrists in cold water to reduce swelling and pressure on the nerves in the wrist. To stretch the carpal tunnel, crouch down and gently press the palms of the hands flat on the floor.

When you rest, make sure you elevate your hands and forearms on pillows, and take extra care when handling hot liquids, especially when you first wake up and the symptoms and numbness are at their worst.

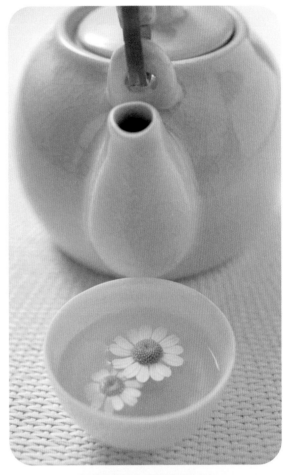

CHAMOMILE MOUTHWASH
Infuse 2 teaspoons of chamomile in freshly boiled water for 10 minutes; strain, cool, and rinse around mouth for a minute, then spit out.

> **WARNING If you have severe swelling that doesn't go down, together with a headache, contact your doctor or midwife, as this could be a sign of preeclampsia.**

Emotional Issues

Pregnancy is one of the greatest changes that you are likely to undergo in your life. In addition to all the physical transformations taking place, there are many changing factors in your life that can affect you emotionally and may cause you to feel anxious or depressed or to have sleepless nights.

Anxiety

Whether this is your first or your fourth pregnancy, it is only natural to worry. What's important is that you not allow natural concerns that can motivate you to have the best, healthiest, and most natural pregnancy possible to turn into fruitless and negative anxiety.

If you find that you are anxious a good deal of the time, you should use some of the relaxation techniques on pages 36–9, while eating a nutritious, healthy diet (see pages 42–63) and getting plenty of exercise.

Talking to your friends and partner about your concerns and/or joining a prenatal childbirth class can help to allay your worries. However, if you still feel anxious, some of the following natural remedies may well help.

What to do

When you are anxious, you hold your breath and your chest is tight. Take your mind off your worries by focusing on your breathing. As you breathe in, slow your breath to the count of three, then slowly breathe out to the count of four. Repeat this exercise until you feel your body and your ribcage start to relax. You can accentuate the calming effects of this breathing exercise if you visualize your in-breath as a vivid blue color, and the out-breath as a glittering gold. You'll find that as you relax and breathe more deeply, the breathing will move from shallow breaths in your upper chest through lower chest and then to the belly, giving your body the rich oxygen it needs.

As you feel your levels of anxiety rising, take a couple of drops of the Bach Rescue Remedy to help you relax. Alternatively, a couple of drops of chamomile, lavender, rose, mandarin, or sandalwood essential oil in a warm bath can be very soothing.

Drinking calming herbal teas, such as chamomile or lemon balm, throughout the day can also help to keep anxiety at bay.

Sleeplessness

Paradoxically, many pregnant women—despite being completely exhausted at bedtime—have difficulty sleeping. They may have trouble getting to sleep in the first place, or they may be awakened by the baby's movements or by needing to go to the toilet and then be unable to fall asleep again. However, adequate sleep and rest are important if you are to be ready to cope with the demands of a new baby.

What to do

Before bedtime, create an environment that is conducive to sleep. So avoid stimulating activities, such as the computer, telephone calls, or hectic television shows. Instead, turn to quieter, more relaxing activities, such as reading, taking a candlelit bath (add a couple of drops of lavender oil), or listening to relaxing music. Make sure that you are not so relaxed

greenfile

Consider hypnotherapy or counseling if your anxiety levels are ruining the enjoyment of your baby's imminent arrival.

WARNING A certain amount of anxiety during pregnancy is natural, but if you suspect that your levels of stress and anxiety are adversely affecting you or your baby, or if depression persists, talk to your doctor or midwife.

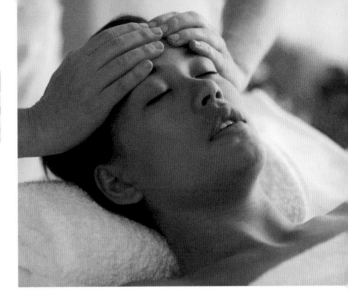

in the bath that you fall asleep, and always take fire safety precautions if using candles.

The common tradition of having a hot milky drink at bedtime is based on scientific fact. Milk contains calcium, which helps to combat insomnia and relax muscles. So a cup of warm milk with a sprinkling of cinnamon added can be very beneficial if taken just before you retire for the night. If you're not fond of cow's milk, then chamomile, passionflower, or lime blossom herbal tea as a bedtime drink can be effective in helping you to fall asleep.

Depression

There are many reasons why you may have odd moments of depression while pregnant, even if you do not suffer from the condition at other times. Firstly, you probably realize that hormonal changes can affect both your physical and your emotional state, but did you know that depression can also result from nutritional deficiencies and dehydration? There is also the more obvious emotional upset caused by the reemergence of old fears and new concerns about coping. Nutritional deficiencies and dehydration can be easily avoided or rectified by following a healthy-eating regime and drinking plenty of water. Emotional causes of depression can be helped by a holistic approach.

What to do

Numerous studies have shown that regular exercise reduces the number of depressive episodes and anxiety attacks and increases emotional stability. So get out there doing whichever activity appeals most, whether it's swimming, walking, yoga, tai chi, or ballroom dancing!

When you're depressed, you breathe six times faster than when you're not, so if you're feeling low, try the breathing exercises for calming anxiety (see page 132).

Massage is proven to alleviate depression, as it stimulates the release of the body's natural painkillers (endorphins) and reduces levels of the stress hormones, cortisol and norepinephrine. A regular massage, or even a back and shoulder rub by your partner, can be relaxing and a great bulwark against depression.

Certain essential oils work very quickly on your nervous system and can be effective against temporary episodes of depression. Orange blossom, mandarin, grapefruit, rose, and lavender oils are all effective. Use a couple of drops of oil added to a bath, in a vaporizer, or blended with a carrier oil for aromatherapy massage. Complementary therapies such as flower essences, herbalism, reiki, acupuncture, hypnotherapy, and homeopathy all report good results for treating depression. Also consult a nutritionist, as nutritional deficiencies are often a cause of hormonal imbalance.

greenfile

Although governmental agencies and conventional health professionals have approved the artificial sweetener aspartame as safe for pregnant women, many holistic practitioners advise that women avoid it during pregnancy because it is linked to food allergies, sensitivities, and depression. Check food and drink labels—aspartame is widely used in diet colas and low-sugar or low-calorie foods.

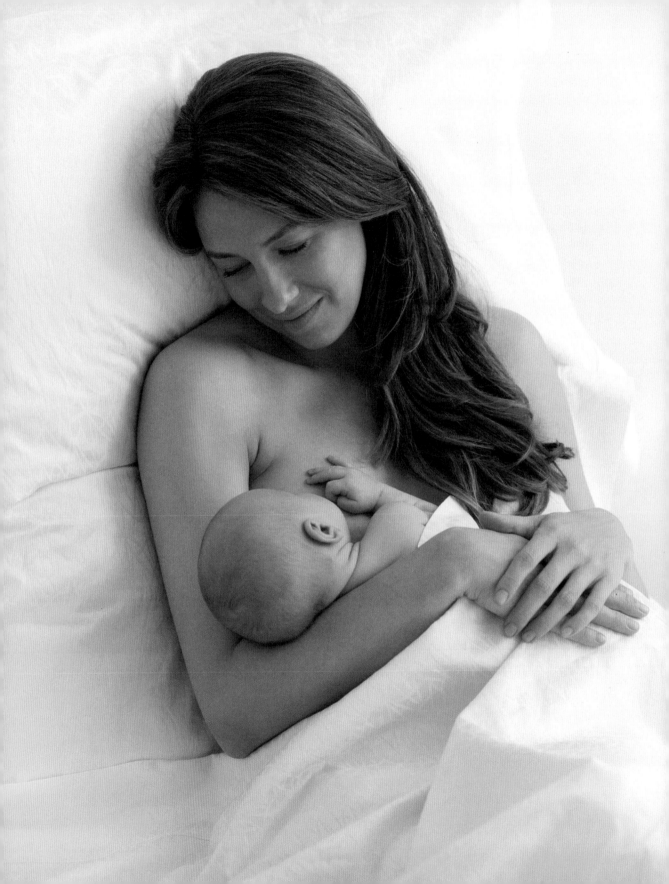

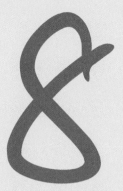

Natural Birth Options

You have come all the way through your pregnancy choosing the greener, more natural options for you and your baby. Now, as you near the date for the birth and the start of a new phase in your life, it's time to make some important decisions about the type of birthing experience that you would most like to have.

Certainly, there is no right or wrong way to give birth. At home? In a hospital? With or without pain relief? These are the kinds of questions that will be running through your mind as you approach full term, yet only you can know what feels right for you. However, if you acquaint yourself fully with all the birthing options available, you stand a better chance of choosing the setting and style that best resonates with you and your beliefs.

The following pages give you the lowdown on what to expect when you go into labor (see page 136), so you can start to form an idea about whether you might want a home birth (see page 140). If you lean toward a hospital birth, there are ways to make the experience as green and natural as possible and to avoid many of the routine medical interventions (see pages 143–6).

Finally, let's look slightly farther ahead. We'll assume that you've had a wonderful birth experience and that you and your new family are settling back in to life at home. A few tips about those early postpartum days may prove useful (see page 152).

Childbirth

By the end of a pregnancy most mothers are eagerly anticipating the arrival of their baby, but very few look forward to the labor. In part, this is because the unknown is always frightening; and, irrespective of whether it's your first or your fourth child, every delivery is different.

Nonetheless, while no one can really prepare you for what you are about to experience, if you have prepared well for the birth and have a relaxed and positive approach, you will fare better than if you are overtired or anxious.

During your prenatal care you should have been encouraged to think about the kind of birth experience you would like and even to formulate a birth plan (see page 89). By the same token, you should also have been warned that things do not always go to plan and that you have the right to change your mind.

Women who have very set ideas about how their birth will progress can feel that they have let themselves down if things do not go according to plan. This is a great shame, and such unyielding views put an unrealistic burden upon the mother (and baby).

There is no wrong or right way to have a baby. So long as the baby is not put at any risk, you do whatever you have to do to get through the birth the best way possible. In the United States a majority of women have epidural anesthesia during labor, although many choose a natural delivery instead. So long as your baby is safe, there is no extra merit in giving birth without pain relief unless it is what you truly want to do.

If you find the labor very painful or unbearable, don't feel afraid to ask for pain relief. You have not failed in any way, and there is no shame attached. After all, it is not a competition. Yet for those who prefer to experience the whole birthing process naturally, I can vouch for the fact that it is a wondrous experience. None of us knows how we are going to react in the face of pain and the unknown, so just keep an open mind.

Giving Birth

Labor is usually classified into three stages. How long it takes from start to finish varies considerably from individual to individual, and, in the main, there is very little that you can do to affect the duration of the birth. It has to be said that a fit, relaxed, and healthy woman tends to have an easier time of it, simply because she has more stamina and physical resources to draw upon. However, sometimes, the most slothful of women deliver in a matter of minutes while the athlete finds herself pushing hours later. There is no rhyme or reason for it. Nonetheless, whatever the duration of labor, we all follow the same stages of the process.

First Stage: Labor

Early labor stage This is when the cervix softens and starts to dilate to the first 1½ in (4 cm). You may have a "bloody show" during this stage (the name given to the plug of mucus that was guarding the entrance of the cervix). Some women's waters break before or during the first part of labor, and these fluids (from the amniotic sac) serve as a useful lubrication. Don't worry if your waters don't break at the outset; they will go in good

greenfile

Do what feels natural and comfortable to you. However, correct breathing, walking, kneeling, standing, or sitting in different positions are all known to help to ease the pain of contractions. Try to relax fully between contractions and take lots of fluids—sports drinks and fruit juices if allowed, otherwise water and/or ice cubes.

LABOR BAG FOR THE HOSPITAL

Have your bag ready from around 36 weeks, in case you need to head out the door in a hurry! Suggested contents:

Clothes for you during labor and after birth, including bathrobe and nursing bra, slippers, and socks (your feet can get cold during labor)

Clothes for baby (including a bodysuit or sleeper, socks, blanket, hat, outdoor clothes to travel home) and diapers

Toiletries, including moisturizer, lip balm containing aloe vera and vitamin E, and massage oil

Hair bands or scrunchies, if appropriate

Hot water bottle or wheat bag

Hand mirror for watching head crowning

Approved flower essences, aromatherapy oils, or homeopathic remedies

Scented candles and relaxing music

TENS machine, with batteries, if appropriate (see page 147)

Food for you and your birth partner

Camera/camcorder and list of telephone numbers of friends

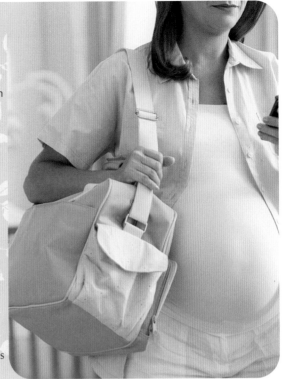

time. The caregiver may offer to rupture the membrane artificially for you—this is your choice (see page 143).

At the beginning, contractions can be 10–20 minutes apart, lasting up to 30 seconds, or they may be every five minutes and lasting a minute or more. Although it may seem like no small achievement to you, sad to say, this is still called the early labor, or sometimes learn-to-labor, phase.

PROGRESS CHECK

To check how far you have progressed in your labor, the caregiver will insert her fingers into your vagina to check the softness (effacement) and openness (dilation) of the cervix. This examination should not be painful, although many women report discomfort. During the early (latent) stage of labor you may dilate up to 1½ in (4 cm), during the active stage from 1½–2¾ in (4–7 cm); during transition you will dilate from 2¾–4 in (7–10 cm). Once you are fully dilated, the baby is ready to be born.

Before you head to the hospital (when contractions are 3–4 minutes apart, although you should be guided by your caregiver), you can help to ease contractions by walking around or taking a warm bath.

Active or hard labor starts once you've passed the 1½ in (4 cm) dilation point. During this phase, your baby descends farther into the pelvis and you become fully dilated (4in [10cm]).

You should now be doing the breathing and relaxation exercises that you learned at your prenatal classes. However, I hesitate to say that you "should" be doing anything, since, although midwives and caregivers report that this works to good effect, you are mistress of your own destiny at this point, and "should" really doesn't come into it.

Transition Dilation from 1½–4 in (4–10 cm) can take a matter of minutes or hours. For many women, this is the hardest part of the delivery. It's known as the transition, or advanced active, phase of labor.

Contractions are intensely painful and seem interminable. At the end of this stage, you may experience a lot of pressure against your lower back, perineum, and rectum, and the desire to push down and expel the baby is at its strongest.

At this point, some women, myself included, experience a serene moment of tranquillity, akin to the calm before the storm, as the body prepares itself for the big push.

Second Stage: Delivery

Pushing You may get a renewed burst of energy at this point in your labor, or you may simply feel exhausted

BIRTHING POSITIONS

No longer are women expected to lie on their back on a bed to deliver a baby. There are many options available now, both for a home and hospital delivery. Getting into the best position during labour and birth can speed up the process considerably and make you more comfortable throughout. Why not try:

Kneeling on hands and knees

Sitting or reclining (on a birthing stool, the toilet, a birthing ball or reclining against the side of a bed or birth rail)

Squatting (supported or free-standing)

Upright or standing

Side-lying (particularly beneficial for resting during a long labour)

Keeping your mouth and jaw relaxed during breathing helps to keep your vaginal muscles relaxed, too.

and just want the whole business over and done with. Unfortunately, whatever your feelings, you have no choice but to work quite hard now.

Once you feel pushing urges, your baby should be born within a couple of hours. Second-time mothers may even deliver their baby within ten minutes of feeling the urge to push.

As you push with each contraction, you'll feel the baby move forward and then slide back a little. Don't be discouraged—it's quite natural and, in fact, good for the baby and your expanding vagina.

Crowning As the head starts to crown (when the widest part of the head is still visible after a contraction ends), you'll experience extreme pressure in your bottom, often described as a burning feeling, and many women report a sensation of tearing at the perineum. This is rarely the case, and the caregiver will be applying pressure to the area to reduce the risk of tears or need for an episiotomy (see page 145).

Delivery As your baby's head emerges, you may well feel a burning sensation in your vagina, and you may be told to stop pushing at this point to avoid tearing. Once the head is out, your baby will turn

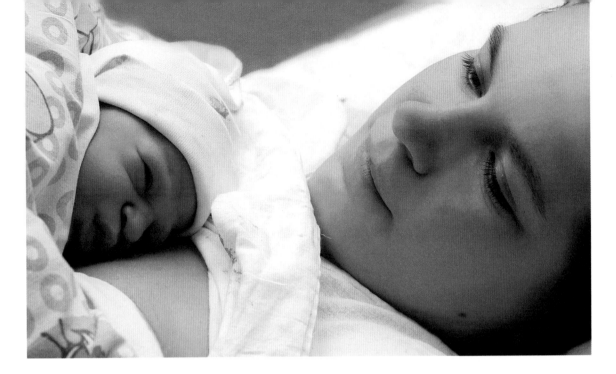

to one side, the shoulders will come out, and, finally, the rest of the body will follow. The relief and elation are immense.

Holding your baby What happens next varies, depending on where you have your baby and your personal preferences. Sometimes the baby is placed on your abdomen directly after the birth. On other occasions, the baby is checked and wrapped before being placed in your arms. The caregiver will assess your baby using the Apgar scale (see page 141).

Third Stage: Delivering the Placenta

At some point shortly after your baby has been born, you will be asked to expel the placenta. As your caregiver places a hand on your abdomen, she'll ask you to push again. You may feel slight cramps, but the euphoria at having your baby usually tempers this.

It is important that your uterus contract at this stage to minimize bleeding. If your caregiver suspects you're losing too much blood, she may massage your abdomen vigorously to encourage the uterus to contract, or you may be given an injection that has the same effect.

AFTER PAINS

"After pains" is the name given to contractions that occur after you have given birth. They are caused by your uterus shrinking back down to its pre-pregnancy size and shape, which usually takes around 15 days.

After pains are not a cause for concern, but they can cause discomfort or even pain. Although some women are not affected, those who are notice that contractions are most intense in the first few days after giving birth. You may also notice them more when you breast-feed. This happens because the uterus is still sensitive to the oxytocin released while nursing.

Some people believe that after pains are negligible with a first baby and that they increase after each subsequent baby, although this is not always the case.

Comfort measures include placing warm packs or a hot-water bottle on your abdomen, gently massaging your abdomen and visualizing a stream of energy flowing through your uterus, down your legs to your toes.

If after pains are persistently severe after a week or so, consult your doctor to eliminate any other problems, such as infection.

Home Births

It comes as no surprise that women have been having babies at home for centuries. What's less well known is that research now shows that if you are a low-risk pregnant woman attended by a trained caregiver, a home birth is perfectly safe. In fact, some advocates of home birth would argue that home births are safer in terms of the lowered risk of infection, the need for intervention, and maternal hemorrhaging.

So if you have a loving and safe home environment and your obstetric team evaluate you as a low-risk pregnancy, then this could be the most natural option for you. Unfortunately, if you are expecting twins, if your baby is in the breech position, or if you're a first-time mother aged over 35, your doctor/midwife team are less likely to sanction a home birth, although it's not impossible to proceed.

However, one important consideration to take into account when making a decision about a home birth is how close the hospital facilities are, just in case something were to go wrong and you need to be transferred for an emergency cesarean delivery or resuscitation of the baby. If you live a long way from medical facilities, this could influence your decision to have a home birth, and it might also affect the agreement of your attending midwife.

These risks have to be weighed against the undoubted benefits of being relaxed and comfortable in your own home environment with your loved ones (and possibly children) around you—what could be more natural!

Labor and Birth

Let us assume that you fit all the criteria and you're having your baby at home. You should have on hand all the necessary supplies that your midwife has recommended when your labor starts. Your midwife will join you at your home once the contractions are approximately 3–4 minutes apart. She will probably encourage you to walk and stand as much as possible

GREEN GOODY BAG
Make sure you have readily on hand a selection of your favorite green goodies. Suggestions include:

Hot-water bottle or wheat bag

Ice cubes

Lip balm (containing aloe vera and vitamin E)

Hand mirror for watching head crowning

Massage oil

Approved flower essences and aromatherapy oils

Approved botanical/herbal or homeopathic remedies

Scented candles

Relaxing music

Beanbag

Warm socks

Birth ball, stool, or pool, if appropriate

TENS machine, with batteries, if appropriate
(see page 147)

to increase dilation. She will regularly check your dilation, effacement, urine, blood pressure, pulse, and temperature. She will also listen to the baby's heart rate using a Doppler stethoscope or a fetoscope (trumpet).

Apart from these periodic checks, you are free to move around, assume any position that's comfortable, or rest, as you wish. If you have had a birthing pool set up at home, you may spend as much time in the water as you like. You can use approved herbal tinctures, acupressure, flower essences, homeopathic remedies, massage, candles, music, and supplements to your heart's content—your midwife may well encourage this. Some midwives are even trained in providing holistic remedies to help ease the pain and speed up labor.

Your partner, friends, or relatives who are with you are at liberty to be as involved as they want to be, or as much as feels right for you. A massage from your partner can be hugely relaxing and beneficial, as can a cool cloth wiped over your face. Sometimes, standing with your arms around your partner's neck and pushing down can be helpful; and it, too, is very inclusive.

Unless there are signs that your baby is becoming distressed, or the labor is progressing very slowly, you will be encouraged to push only when you feel like it. Home-birth midwives often suggest that you try pushing while bent over on your hands and knees. This is a comfortable position and can sometimes speed up labor. Others may bring a birthing stool for you to try.

A trained caregiver may offer you a perineal massage when the baby's head is resting on the perineal floor. Some believe this reduces the need for an episiotomy. As the head crowns (see page 138), you might like to ask if someone can hold a mirror for you so you can see the first glimpse of your new baby.

As soon as the baby is born, she will be placed on your abdomen or chest. Some midwives suction the baby's nose and mouth and dry her before passing her to you. Your partner may be invited to cut the baby's cord. The baby is assessed using the Apgar scale (see below).

THE APGAR TEST
This test, given by the midwife, assesses the health of your newborn baby at one and five minutes after the birth.

It checks your baby's Appearance, Pulse, Grimace, Activity and Respiration.

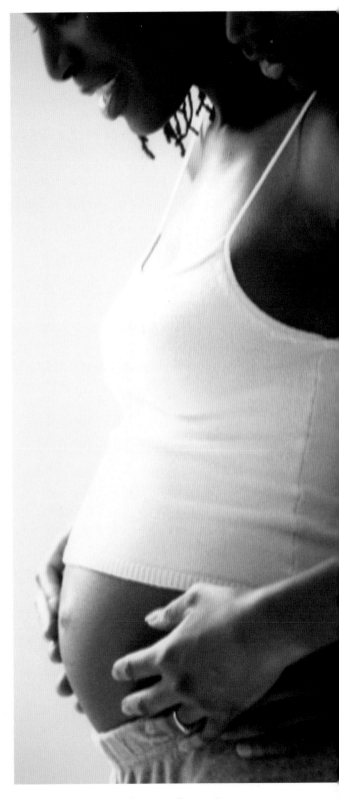

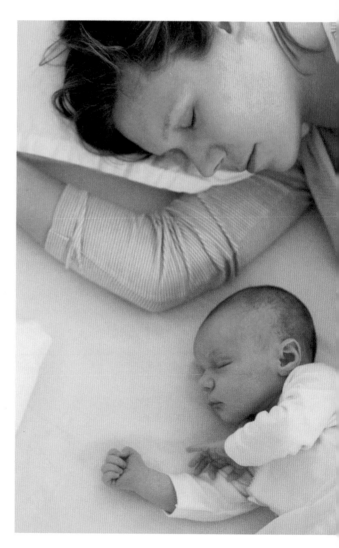

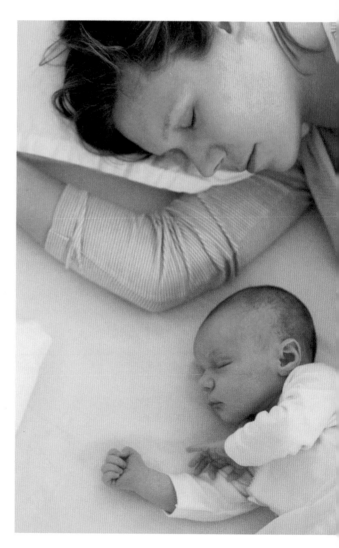

Your midwife may use nipple stimulation to speed up your labor. A hot shower may also be suggested.

Women who deliver their baby at home rarely require suturing (stitches).

After the Birth

At a home birth, the midwife prefers for the placenta to be expelled naturally, and this can take anywhere up to an hour. The baby will probably be put to your breast, as this stimulates the nipples, which in turn increases uterine contractions and so helps to expel the placenta. The midwife may also strongly massage your abdomen to encourage its expulsion. If, however, there is no sign of the placenta separating, you will be given an injection to make this happen.

Once the placenta has been checked to make sure it is intact and you have been examined for tears and lacerations and treated, if necessary, you will then be left alone with your new baby and your partner, friends, or family. This is a wonderful moment that you will cherish for a lifetime.

About an hour or so later, the midwife will return to give your baby a vitamin K injection, if agreed, or oral medication if not. Your baby will also receive eyedrops immediately after the birth to prevent any eye infections. The midwife will complete a neonatal examination of your baby and also check on your progress. You are then left in peace in the comfort of your own home with your new family, but you can, of course, call your midwifery team at any time if you have any concerns or worries, about either yourself or your baby.

Most mothers who retain their placenta for disposal choose to bury it (or "plant" it) in the garden. It's even been known for mothers to put colored inks on it and to take a print—one mother told me that with the umbilical cord hanging down, the print looked like the Tree of Life. Occasionally, a woman chooses to eat the placenta (most often fried in butter but occasionally raw) to get the nutrients.

If you choose to dispose of your placenta yourself, it is perfectly safe to keep it in the freezer while you decide what you'd like to do.

THE PLACENTA—YOUR OPTIONS

After checking that the placenta is intact, the midwife will seal it in a plastic bag and take it away to dispose of it, usually by incineration. If you wish, you can keep the placenta to dispose of yourself; however, you should check your state law regarding its disposal.

Greener Birth Options

Since you have chosen to read this book, it is highly likely that you have followed a natural, green, and optimum health approach to your pregnancy, which is sure to offer your baby the very best start in life.

Nonetheless, as you reach the last weeks of your pregnancy, despite your best efforts to date, certain unavoidable circumstances could increase the chances of medical intervention during the birth. Should you find yourself in one of these out-of-the-ordinary situations, here are some natural suggestions for averting the need for medical help.

Breech Position

If your baby is in a breech position (head under your ribs and bottom in your pelvis), after 34–36 weeks, there is a good chance that your medical team will suggest a cesarean delivery. Vaginal breech deliveries are rarely offered for breech babies now, but if your baby is not successfully turned and you want a vaginal delivery, it would be sensible to discuss this with your obstetrician or midwife, who can advise on the availability of delivery staff who have appropriate experience. Some doctors advise an epidural for every woman having a vaginal delivery breech birth, but this is not strictly necessary.

The external turning of your baby can be effective, but it is not without risks and should be attempted only by an experienced midwife or physician, who will monitor the baby's heartbeat as he is being turned.

The natural way

In order to avoid having to make these decisions about this kind of medical intervention, there are several natural procedures you might like to consider that may assist in turning your baby before the birth.

There has been a suggestion that spending 15 minutes every two hours of the waking day in the knee-chest position will help the baby to turn (known as Elkin's maneuver).

There is some evidence that hypnotherapy may be useful, although only one study has looked at this. Acupuncture has been suggested as an effective therapy for turning breech babies, and the results of a formal study are awaited.

Older midwives recommend massaging your belly with almond oil for ten minutes while lying on your back with your hips higher than your head. Before you start this regime, ask your midwife which way your baby is most likely to turn so that you can massage in the correct direction.

A Canadian study has shown that classical music may be able to turn a breech baby. Headphones were placed on the mother's lower abdomen, and calming classical music was played for an hour each day over a five-day period. Often the baby turns toward the source of the music.

Finally, there is anecdotal evidence to suggest that swimming may help a baby to turn. There is no scientific explanation for this, but some people believe it's due to the double buoyancy of the mother and baby in the water.

Breaking Waters

Some doctors and midwives perform artificial rupture of membranes (ARM or breaking the waters) to speed up labor if it's progressing slowly. This procedure can be done during an internal examination. A midwife or doctor makes a small break in the membranes around your baby, using either an amnihook (a long thin probe, which looks a little like a fine crochet hook) or an amnicot (a medical glove with a pricked end on one of the fingers). This procedure often works when the cervix feels soft and ready for labor to start.

However, ARM does not always work, and once your waters have been broken, your baby could be at risk of infection. Moreover, it shortens labor by only about an hour, and it does tend to increase pain, as the baby's head is now directly on the cervix. This can necessitate more pain relief and possibly more interventions.

Birthing in water is a good way to minimize the risk of ARM, because the pressure of the water often helps to do this naturally. There is debate among midwives about whether a baby should be allowed to be born without the membranes' breaking. Some believe it can cushion the head through the birth canal and poses no danger to the baby. Others believe ARM is necessary to check that there is no meconium (waste from the first bowel movement) in the amniotic fluid, which can indicate that the baby is in distress.

Monitoring

In hospitals, your baby's heartbeat is generally monitored throughout labor, so that any problems with the baby are able to be detected at the earliest possible moment. This usually involves attaching you to a monitor via a belt or pads placed on the abdomen; the baby's heartbeat is then recorded on screen. The other, less common form of monitoring involves placing an electrode on the baby's scalp via the vagina.

Either method is restrictive. If you want to move freely, you will have to ask your attendant to monitor intermittently rather than continuously. Alternatively, you can request that your baby's heart rate be monitored using an electronic stethoscope (Doppler) or a fetoscope, just as it would be if you were having a home delivery.

Induction

If the birth of your baby is more than two weeks overdue, your medical team will probably want to induce you. The methods of induction of labor normally offered by medical staff are membrane sweeping, which is a drug-free intervention (see right), prostaglandin gel, or pessaries, which are inserted into the vagina (or occasionally given orally), artificial rupture of the membranes (see pages 143–4), or an oxytocin drip, which is given in the synthetic form of Pitocin (in the U.S.) or Syntocinon (in Britain).

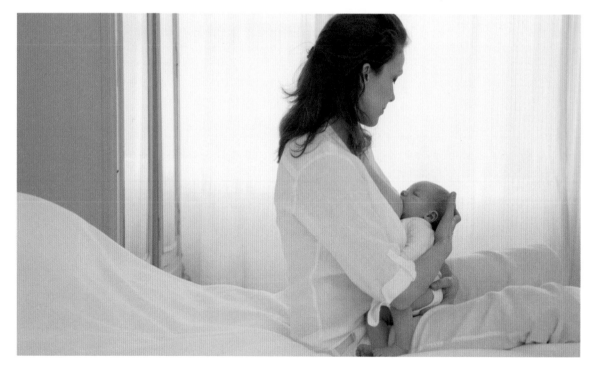

The natural way

Holistic therapies, such as homeopathy, acupuncture, reflexology, aromatherapy, flower essences, and herbal remedies, have all been known to give good results in starting labor.

Many traditional self-help methods for inducing labor are still used in traditional societies. The evidence for their efficacy tends to be anecdotal, but support for the following methods persists:

- Lots of moderate exercise
- Sexual intercourse
- Eating spicy food, such as curry
- Taking a car ride down a bumpy road
- Nipple stimulation for at least an hour (you could use a breast pump rather than doing it manually)
- Eating lots of fresh pineapple
- Drinking raspberry leaf or cumin tea
- Adding a few drops of clary sage and jasmine essential oil to a bath

WARNING Herbal, aromatherapy, and homeopathic self-help measures are extremely potent and are dangerous if used without the advice of a trained practitioner.

- Drinking 3 teaspoons of castor oil mixed in a glass of orange juice. (Note: castor oil can give you cramps and diarrhea—use with great caution)
- Taking herbal remedies blue cohosh or goldenseal
- Taking the homeopathic remedy Caulophyllum 30c and Gelsemium

Note: It is worth bearing in mind that complementary therapies and self-help measures to induce labor are still an intervention, albeit usually a gentler one than hospital induction. Nonetheless, you are interfering with your body's natural rhythms and ability to give birth at the right time for you, so you should think through why exactly you are doing this. If it's about avoiding a hospital induction, then a natural route to starting labor can be just as effective.

Tearing and Episiotomy

When your vagina does not stretch enough, or the baby comes out too quickly, a tear in the perineum can occur. If, during the labor, your doctor or midwife suspects this may happen to you, they will probably suggest an episiotomy (a small cut from the vagina toward the anus) under local anesthetic. The cut, or a tear, is then sutured (stitched) after the birth.

There are those in the holistic field who believe that it is preferable to tear naturally rather than to have an episiotomy, since a natural tear is thought to heal more quickly.

The natural way

Undoubtedly, it is better if you can avoid tearing or an episiotomy altogether, and there are several measures you can take to help prevent this.

Perineal massage during your pregnancy is often recommended as a way to prepare your vaginal canal for birth and to prevent tearing, although the evidence suggests this helps with superficial tearing only. Vitamin E oil and almond oil with chamomile or calendula added are excellent oils for perineal massage.

Lovemaking is another good way to tone and prepare your uterus and vaginal muscles for the birth.

During the birth, some midwives use oil poured on the perineal area to lubricate and prevent tearing. There are also precautions you can take to help yourself. As the baby's head begins to emerge, you'll feel a stretching or stinging sensation in your vagina. At this point, try to resist pushing and adopt rapid, short, panting breaths or blowing, so that the baby exits slowly. Most midwives agree that taking time at this stage is the best way to prevent tearing—they may also encourage you to lie on your left side, as this seems to be the optimum position to deliver slowly and without tearing.

Recently, midwives and doulas (see page 150) have started to recommend that you draw your legs together and rock your hips from side to side, as if rocking your baby, at this crowning stage of the birth to avoid delivering the baby too quickly, which causes tearing.

Cesarean

Once the effects of the anesthetic have worn off, you can experience some pain after a cesarean section. Many midwives recommend mild analgesics to take the edge off the pain so you can nurse your baby.

The natural way

Midwives encourage breast-feeding after a cesarean, because it produces endorphins, which will ease the pain. When breast-feeding, try placing a pillow over your stomach to support the baby and protect the sore area.

Be careful not to pull or strain your abdominal or stomach muscles. Sleeping on your side, supported by large pillows may help. Flower and homeopathic remedies can bring gentle relief from both physical and emotional problems after a cesarean section. If you feel weepy, which is common, try Arnica 6c or Rescue Remedy to help stabilize your emotions.

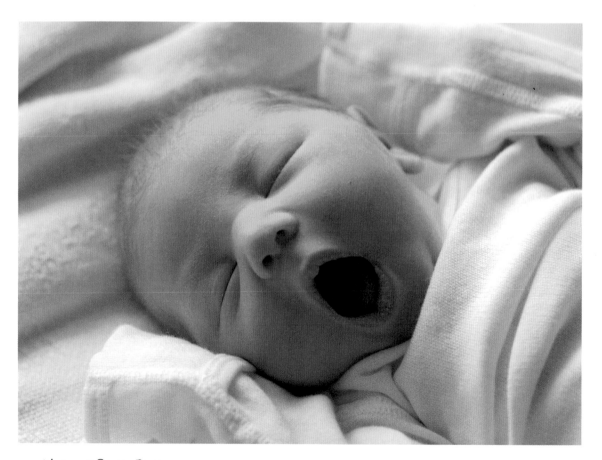

Natural Pain Relief

None of us can know how we are going to cope with the pain of labor, especially if this is a first baby. Yet knowledge is power, and if you are aware of the various methods of pain relief that are available, you can approach the coming birth feeling confident and positive about how you will deal with the pain.

If you are keen to avoid the use of conventional drugs or anesthetics, the following natural pain relief methods not only are effective but can also help you to enjoy a natural and wondrous birth.

Acupuncture

Whether at home or in a medical setting, an acupuncture practitioner in attendance at the birth can be very helpful for managing painful contractions and backache. Needles may be inserted in the ear in order to trigger the release of endorphins, the body's natural painkillers, and it takes about half an hour for the buildup to become effective. Acupoints on your lower back and spine may also be stimulated

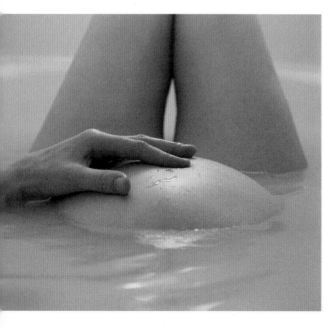

in order to ease back pain and those on the hand to make the contractions more effective.

TENS

A TENS (transcutaneous electrical nerve stimulation) machine works along principles similar to acupuncture but can be administered either yourself or by your birthing partner. Electrodes in pads are attached to acupoints on your lower back, and a pulsed electric current blocks pain messages from the cervix and uterus to the brain. The current is controlled by a hand-held control device, so you can move around with ease, increasing or reducing the intensity of the current with the contractions.

TENS seems to work best and give you the most effective pain relief if you start using it at the very beginning of your labor. It takes about an hour for your body to respond to the electrical impulses by releasing endorphins, so start using it as soon as you begin to get contractions or backache. Start with the controls at their lowest settings, and turn them up gradually as your contractions or the back pain gets stronger. Use the boost button at the peak of contractions.

Warmth and Water

Warmth from a wrapped hot-water bottle or wheat bag placed on your back, tummy, or groin can help to relieve the pain of labor.

Taking a warm bath is known to make contractions more bearable, which is why some women book a complete water birth. And there is clinical evidence to support the increasing number of women who opt for this birth experience. A British study by the Oxford Centre for Health Care Research and Development in 2001, showed that the need for pain-relieving narcotics and epidurals was significantly lower when women labor in a birthing pool.

In light of this and other research, in September 2007, Britain's National Institute for Health and Clinical Excellence recommended that all expectant mothers be offered a water birth for the safest form of pain relief. It stated that birthing pools are second only to epidurals in alleviating pain.

Some women view a birthing pool as a form of pain relief that can be tried before resorting to other medical alternatives, if necessary. In fact, you can quite easily take gas and air (see page 149) while in a birthing pool if you should wish to combine the two.

Breathing

Focusing on your breathing is an effective and safe way of getting through each contraction.

At the beginning of the contraction, take a deep breath in through your nose.

As you breathe out through your mouth, visualize the pain and tension ebbing away from your body and actively relax.

You don't have to breathe too deeply—just concentrate on keeping a good rhythm going.

Repeat again and again, keeping your face, jaw, and mouth soft. Concentrate fully on your breathing as the contraction builds up, and as it fades away.

When the contraction is over, relax.

Massage

Since time immemorial, massage has been one of the simplest yet most effective ways to relieve pain during labor.

You can tell your birth partner or midwife where and how you'd like to be massaged; slow, rhythmical movements tend to ease tension, and firmer strokes can stimulate you when your energies are flagging, especially during a lengthy labor.

Hypnotherapy

Self-hypnosis techniques have proven so successful in helping to control the pain of labor that it is now a recognized birthing option known as HypnoBirthing (or the Mongan Method).

A course of prenatal lessons teaches you simple but powerful self-hypnosis techniques to induce feelings of relaxation and peace during labour and birth. The aim is to help release any fears and anxieties that naturally affect many pregnant women, whether they are facing their first experience of labor or have had traumatic births previously. The emphasis is very much on the woman staying in control of her own mind and body, rather than feeling helpless and disempowered.

Although the use of hypnosis cannot guarantee a totally pain-free labor, the HypnoBirthing Institute (see Useful Contacts, page 156) offers some impressive statistics on the advantages of this method. For example, out of more than 1,000 American mothers who used the HypnoBirthing method, 72 percent used no pain medication. Only 15.5 percent of mothers using hypnosis had cesarean deliveries, as compared to the national average of 32 percent. The incidence of preterm babies was also significantly lower than the national average.

Aromatherapy

A few drops of lavender essential oil can be added to your massage base oil for additional pain relief and relaxation. Chamomile, bergamot, mandarin, and frankincense essential oils are great for their calming effect and to relieve anxiety.

Clary sage is often recommended to help improve contractions, but this is a very powerful essential oil and should be prepared in advance by a qualified aromatherapy practitioner and used only under his strict guidance.

Flower Essences

Take Bach Rescue Remedy or mimulus flower remedy if you're feeling fearful or have a sense of rising panic. Rescue Remedy and Star of Bethlehem can be helpful if you feel you are struggling. In the latter stages of labor, mugwort flower remedy is said to promote the birthing process, while walnut can help you to adjust to the rapid physical changes your body is experiencing.

Homeopathy

Consult a qualified homeopath before you go into labor. S/he may recommend certain remedies, such as Aconite 6c, for rapid contractions; Pulsatilla 6c for back pain, Belladonna 6c for sciatic pain (radiating down your back into your thighs), or Gelsemium 6c for abdominal cramps.

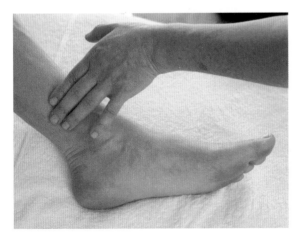

CONVENTIONAL PAIN RELIEF

ANESTHETIC (e.g. epidural) Blocks all pain locally. An epidural is administered by an anesthesiologist via a catheter into your spine, to numb the nerves in your uterus and surrounding muscles.

Disadvantages You cannot walk around, your blood pressure may drop, you may have to be catheterized to pass urine, it can slow labor and increase chances of use of forceps or ventouse for delivery. Also, there's a small risk of your having a severe headache and a very small risk of nerve damage. In larger doses (more than 100 mcg), these drugs may affect your baby's breathing, or make him drowsy.

INHALED ANALGESICS (e.g. gas and air, also known as Entonox) Takes the edge off the pain, rather than completely blocking it out, and is safe for your baby. Breathed in through a mask at the beginning of a contraction.

Disadvantages It may make you feel slightly light-headed or sick and gives you a dry mouth.

NARCOTICS (e.g. meperidine) These opiates help you to relax and offer some—but not total—pain relief. Administered via injection in your thigh or bottom.

Disadvantages It may make you feel drowsy or sick and can cross the placenta, making your baby drowsy or, occasionally, affecting his breathing.

Reflexology

Reflex points on the ankle bones correspond to the uterus and pelvis and can be stimulated to relieve pain and to regulate contractions. During your pregnancy, consult a trained reflexologist, who can instruct you on where to press during labor.

Doulas

There was once a time when women within the immediate and extended family—mothers, sisters, grandmothers, aunts—would be on hand to serve a nurturing role for a new mother, to guide her by experience and help with the practicalities before, during, and after the birth. This is still the case in certain traditional societies, but in the West this tradition has long since passed. However, a relatively new addition to the childbirth team, the professional doula, is reviving this time-honored role.

If you are not confident that you will get the emotional support you need through the birth, the services of a birth doula could be useful.

A doula is a professional trained in birth physiology and the dynamics of childbearing. She offers emotional and practical support to an expectant woman before, during, and after childbirth. A doula believes in "mothering the mother"—enabling a woman to have the most satisfying and empowered time that she can during pregnancy, birth, and the early days as a new mom.

Although trained and experienced in childbirth (the women who become doulas are often health professionals who want to provide additional services and skills to families), not all doulas have given birth themselves. They have a good knowledge and awareness of female physiology, but the doula is not present at the birth in a clinical role—that is the job of the medical staff and/or midwife.

If there are several people providing you with support during the birth (such as your husband or partner and a family member or friend) as well as a doula, make sure that the members of your "team" all communicate well with each other and that each person is clear about what his or her role will be, so you can remain focused on your labor rather than directing them.

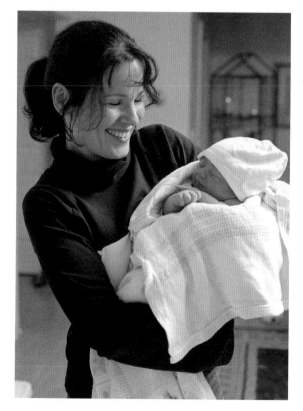

greenfile

"Doula" (pronounced "doola") is a Greek word meaning "woman servant or caregiver."

Birth Doulas

A doula's role is flexible, and she will usually fit in with your specific needs or given situation. In broad terms, she may:

- meet you (and your partner and other children) before the birth
- suggest comfort measures, such as breathing, relaxation, movement, and positioning during the labor
- encourage your partner's active participation in the birth
- nurture, support, and reassure you throughout the birth
- visit you at home once the baby is born

Postnatal Doulas

If you are not able to rely on a good local family and friends support network, you may consider employing a postnatal doula, who specializes in postpartum support.

A postpartum doula's role would usually include both emotional and practical support. She may help with light household duties (laundry, cooking, general straightening-up—you will need to discuss the scope of any domestic duties with her beforehand); she can help with caring for any other children you may have; and she can support breast-feeding (or guide you toward professional breast-feeding support if the need arises.) She also encourages mothers to rest or sleep and will look after your newborn during that time.

Postnatal doulas usually work around three or four hours per day every day or every other day for up to six weeks after the birth (or for a period to be agreed between you).

So if you think that your partner, relatives, or friends can give you the encouragement and support you need during your labor and birth, but that the new baby and housework are getting the better of you,

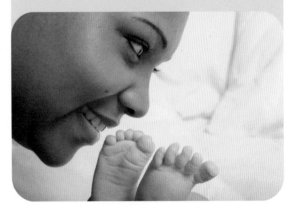

finding the right person

Once you have found a trained doula and established her credentials (see Useful Contacts, page 156), before appointing her ask yourself the following:

Could we spend up to 48 hours together?

Does she listen to me well?

Will she respect my wishes?

Will my partner (or children, if applicable, for a home birth perhaps) like her?

Research shows that having a doula present at a birth helps in these ways:

Shortens first-time labor by an average of 2 hours

Decreases the chance of cesarean section by 50 percent

Decreases the need for pain medication

Helps fathers participate with confidence

Increases success in breast-feeding

perhaps a postpartum doula is a good option for you and will help relieve any stress or anxiety in the early days.

See page 156 for useful contact addresses.

Early Days With Your Baby

So, you have your baby. It's hard to believe that this tiny infant, who has been part of you for so long and whose arrival has been eagerly anticipated, is now here. It is the beginning of a new era, and a period of adjustment will ensue.

However, don't be surprised if the early days after the birth are not quite as you imagined they would be. Sitting cuddling your new baby, surrounded by congratulation cards and flowers, you may find yourself experiencing a range of emotions from elation to sheer terror, indifference to distaste. Some women are lucky enough to sail through the birth, to bond instantly with their baby, and to take the whole business in their stride. But in the early days, most find themselves preoccupied with more basic and pressing problems, such as wanting to urinate without pain, dreading the first bowel movement, and juggling with breast-feeding.

Bonding

Although you may imagine that love for your new baby will be instantaneous, most parents do not feel love at first sight. However, the mothering instinct to

greenfile

A great way to aid bonding is to give your baby a regular massage, which is relaxing and pleasurable for you both. Bathing him, breast- or bottle-feeding, where applicable, or simply cuddling and talking to him also aid the bonding process.

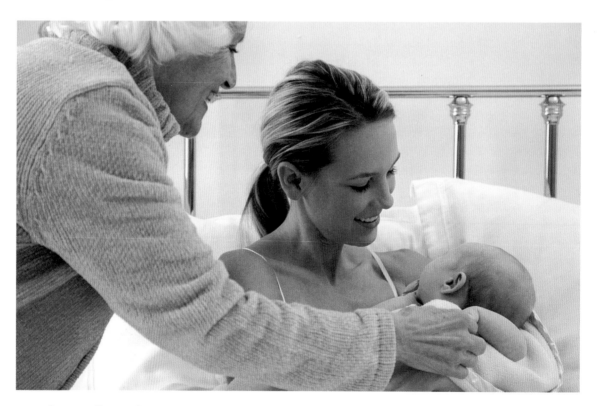

cuddle and protect, if not love, your baby is very strong. In the early days, when you're just getting to know each other, your baby's utter dependence on you will be enough to get you up in the middle of the night in response to his cries.

As time passes and you go about the daily routine of caring for your baby, the bonding process often takes place unnoticed, and it's not until your baby smiles at you and your heart melts that you realize bonding has occurred naturally.

The bonding process may take a little longer if you've had a particularly traumatic birth, if you're depressed, if your baby is in an incubator or needs special care, or if he is handicapped. Some parents simply find it difficult to relate to their baby until he starts to become more responsive and interactive. In fact, there's no single right time to bond with your baby; it's all about building a loving and trusting relationship.

The most important thing to remember is that the bond almost invariably happens sooner or later, but it is less likely to take place if you are tense, depressed, or feeling guilty about your initial reactions. The more you worry about not falling in love, the harder it is to achieve.

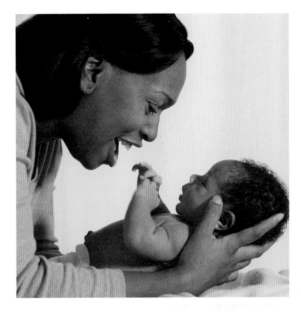

Feeding

How you feed your baby is a highly emotive topic, but it is a decision that you alone can make.

Breast-feeding It is well recognized that breast milk meets your baby's needs perfectly and is digested easily; but your baby won't suffer unduly if you decide

---

greenfile

If you experience discomfort or pain when your milk comes in, there are a few simple green remedies that might help you:

• **If your breasts are engorged, place a cold cabbage leaf (straight from the fridge) inside your bra to ease the pain, and inhale a couple of drops of jasmine oil on a tissue.**

• **The homeopathic remedy Belladonna is recommended, but check with a qualified homeopath for the correct dosage.**

• **Drinking sage tea or taking sage capsules may help reduce engorgement.**

If engorgement develops, and it's too painful to breast-feed, try to empty your breasts yourself using a breast pump or hand expressing methods to prevent mastitis (inflammation of the breasts) from setting in.

Remember, once you've started with full bottle-feeding you can't switch to breast-feeding. Your body will stop producing milk without the stimulation of your baby sucking at the breast.

Despite its being the natural option, breast-feeding can take some time and patience to master. Midwives are excellent at offering help in the early days, but if you don't have this help, you could contact your local branch of the La Leche League, which has breast-feeding counselors who can help you personally (see Useful Contacts, page 156).

to bottle-feed. Feeding your baby should be a pleasure, not a challenge, and it won't be if you breast-feed from a sense of obligation, or bottle-feed while feeling guilty. Don't let anyone make you feel bad about your choice—it's a highly personal issue.

It is scientifically proven that there is no substitute for the colostrum that your breasts produce in the first few days. Breast-feeding your baby will provide him with the valuable antibodies essential for fighting infection in the early months. Even if you feed for a day or two only, it's of benefit to your baby.

Bottle-feeding In some respects, bottle-feeding gives you more freedom and flexibility than breast-feeding: someone else can help with feeds, and fathers often become more involved at an earlier stage with bottle-fed babies. In addition, bottle-fed babies are often able to last longer between feeds, because formula is usually digested more slowly than breast milk. This means that you will probably get longer stretches of uninterrupted sleep in the early days; but bear in mind that a bottle feed takes longer to deliver and you need to prepare the bottles and warm the milk.

Whichever method of feeding you decide upon, remember that the closeness, love, cuddling, and attention that the baby receives at this special time are just as important as the milk that you give him. A relaxed feeding time will provide deep contentment for both you and your baby.

Emotional Adjustment

There is usually help on hand to deal with the physical discomforts. What is less forthcoming is help with the emotional bruises. After all, many new moms feel a bit deflated after the nine-month buildup to the main event. Although delighted to have their baby in their arms, many confess to experiencing feelings of anticlimax after so much hype and expectation. Don't feel guilty about any such emotions—tiredness, surging hormones, and a normal "day-after-the-big-event" ennui are usually at the root of it all. Remember, you are still physically and emotionally vulnerable, so don't attempt to put on a brave face for visitors if you are feeling wretched.

Friends and caregivers may warn you to expect to feel low and weepy on the third or fourth day after the birth. This is commonly known as the "baby blues," and it is characterized by crying spells and feelings of

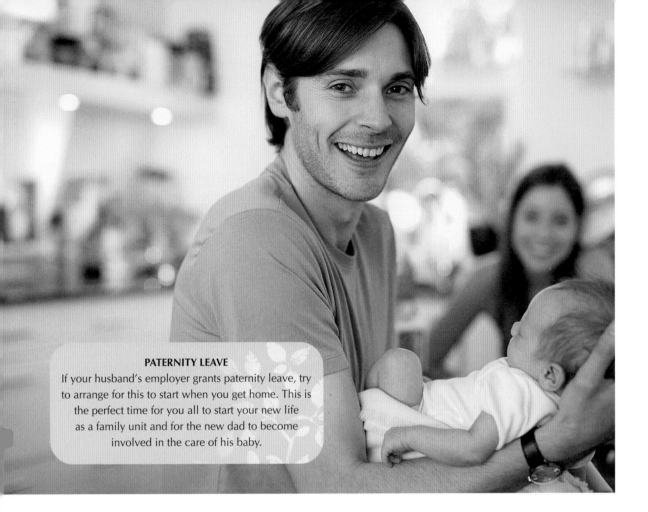

PATERNITY LEAVE
If your husband's employer grants paternity leave, try to arrange for this to start when you get home. This is the perfect time for you all to start your new life as a family unit and for the new dad to become involved in the care of his baby.

inadequacy and exhaustion. It usually passes very quickly, and relaxation, rest, massage, exercise, and good nutrition can hasten the process. However, if these feelings persist, you should talk to your doctor or midwife about it.

Heavy bleeding (see page 154), may lead to anemia, which can also make you feel tired and low. Make sure to inform your healthcare team if you think you may be anemic, and continue to eat iron-rich foods to keep your strength up (see pages 44–5).

The larch, elm, pine, willow, Star of Bethlehem, and crab apple Bach flower remedies are excellent for despondent moments after the birth.

Family Life

Although the father does not have to cope with the physical aftereffects of the birth, he too may well be experiencing mixed emotions. Some men report feeling superfluous and useless during and after the birth, and many lack confidence when it comes to handling their new baby. Conversely, some fathers automatically take on a loving and caring role for the newborn, particularly if the mother is recovering from a hard delivery, and many are surprised and overcome by the depth of their emotions for the new baby. Certainly, the emotional roller coaster that most parents experience in the early days can put a strain on any relationship. Tolerance and understanding are essential during this period of adjustment; and if you can discuss your feelings with one another, you are far more likely to weather any changes that may affect your relationship.

Useful Contacts

A Healthy Start

Lamaze
www.lamaze.org
A nonprofit organization that promotes a natural, healthy, and safe approach to pregnancy, childbirth, and early parenting.

American Massage Therapy Association
www.amtamassage.org

American Meditation Society
www.americanmeditationsociety.org

The American Yoga Association
www.americanyogaassociation.org

Childbirth Connection
www.childbirthconnection.org
Advice to pregnant women and new parents.

Birth International
www.birthinternational.com
Support and resources for midwives, childbirth educators, and expectant parents.

Miscarriage—The American Pregnancy Association
www.americanpregnancy.org/pregnancyloss
Providing support and information for those suffering the effects of pregnancy loss.
Pregnancy Helpline:
1-800-672-2296

Healthy Eating

American Dietetic Association
www.eatright.org
Food and nutritional advice.

The Centers for Disease Control and Prevention (CDC)
www.cdc.gov

US Food and Drug Administration
www.fda.gov

National Institute on Alcohol Abuse and Alcoholism
www.niaaa.nih.gov
See publication Alcohol Alert No 50: Fetal Alcohol Syndrome and the Brain; *and pamphlets and brochures,* Drinking and your Pregnancy.

Alcoholics Anonymous
www.aa.org

Healthy Living

National Stop Smoking
www.smokefree.gov
www.women.smokefree.gov

The Fellowships of Narcotics Anonymous
www.na.org

Safe Cosmetics
www.safecosmetics.org
Advice, campaigns, and DIY recipes for safe, natural cosmetics and toiletries.

US Environmental Protection Agency
www.epa.gov

Consumer Product Safety Commission
www.cpsc.gov
Information on safe products for the home.

The New Parents Guide
www.thenewparentsguide.com
Information on strollers, carriages, and nursery furnishings.

HappyGreenBaby
www.happygreenbaby.com
Eco-friendly and sustainably produced baby clothes and baby gear.

Prenatal Care

The Alliance for the Improvement of Maternity Services (AIMS)
www.aimsusa.org

Lamaze
www.lamaze.org
A nonprofit organization that promotes a natural, healthy and safe approach to pregnancy, childbirth, and early parenting.

Midwives Alliance of North America
www.mana.org

The North American Registry of Midwives
www.narm.org

American Association of Birth Centers (AABC)
www.birthcenters.org

International Confederation of Midwives
www.internationalmidwives.org

Birth Choice
www.birthchoice.net

Water Birth International
www.waterbirth.org

Home Birth USA
www.homebirth-usa.org

Coalition for Improving Maternity Services (CIMS)
www.motherfriendly.org

Remedies and Therapies

American Association of Integrated Medicine
www.aaimedicine.com
Able to help you find an integrated specialist near you.

North American Society of Homeopaths
www.homeopathy.org
The professional association for homeopaths in the USA and Canada.

National Center for Homeopathy
www.nationalcenterforhomeopathy.org

The American Chiropractic Association
www.acatoday.org

American Osteopathic Association
www.osteopathic.org

American Association of Acupuncture and Oriental Medicine
www.aaaomonline.org

Acupuncture/Acupressure Internet Resources
www.holisticmed.com/www/acupuncture.html

The American Herbalists Guild
www.americanherbalistsguild.com

Natural Birth Options

The National Association of Childbirthing Centers (NACC)
www.birthcenters.org
Information about birth centers for parents and healthcare professionals.

The Hypnobirthing Institute
www.hypnobirthing.com
Information and how to find a practitioner.

Doulas of North America
www.dona.org

La Leche League USA
www.lllusa.org
Breastfeeding Helpline:
1-877-4-LALECHE

Index

environmental pollutants
72–5
preparing nursery 76–9
home births 86, 88, 140–1
homeopathy 114–15, 131,
149
hormones, and mood
changes 32
house plants 79
hunger in pregnancy, snacks
31
hypnotherapy 111, 148

immune system, boosting 27
induced birth 90, 95, 144–5
intuition 30–1
ionizers 68
iron 44–5
for fatigue 121
in vegetarian diet 55, 56

labor,
homeopathy in 115, 138,
148
massage during 141
pain relief 147–9
therapies in 105–6, 109,
111–13, 116–17
labor, stages of 144–5
active or hard 137
delivery 138
delivery of placenta 139
early stage 136–7
transition stage 137–8
laundry, green products 71
laxatives, natural 125
Lamaze 98
lead poisoning 76
leg cramps 123
listeriosis 53

magnesium, food sources 48
marijuana 72, 74
massage 39, 105, 126
in labor 141, 143
for new babies 152
for pain relief 148
in pregnancy 38–9
maternity wear 80
meat, in pregnancy 50
medical conditions, and
conception 24
medical herbalism 112–13
meditation 37
membrane sweep, to start
labor 145
microwave ovens 75

midwives 86, 87
and home births 140–2
migraine headaches 130
milk 45
minerals, supplements 23
miscarriage 40–1
molasses 59
monitoring, during labor 144
mood changes 32
morning sickness 69, 120

nailcare 83
narcotics, for pain relief 149
natural birth education
classes 98–9
nursery, preparing 76–9
nutrition 23, 26, 31
healthy eating 43–9
nuts 45, 46

obstetric cholestasis 123
older mothers 96
omega-3 fatty acids 46, 58–9
omega-6 fatty acids 46
opiates 74
organic food 48
osteopathy 103, 131
ovulation 24–5

pain relief,
for the birth 87, 90, 147–9
conventional 149
paint, decorating 76, 77
partners 24, 40, 90
paternity leave 155
peanuts, in pregnancy 52
perineal lubrication 145–6
perineal massage 141
pethidine 149
pilates 27
placenta, delivery of 91, 139,
142
Polarity therapy 126
pollutants, environmental 72–5
postnatal mothers, doulas for
151
therapies for 102–3, 105–6,
109–12, 115–17
poultice, for back pain 126
pre-conceptual health 22–5
preeclampsia 131
pregnancy,
male reactions to 32–3
therapies in 102–3, 105,
109–12, 115–17
prenatal care 85–99
birth plans 89–91

check-ups 92–5
choosing 86–8
classes 98–9
screening and testing 96–7
prescription drugs, and
conception 24
protein, in vegetarian diet 47,
54–6
pushing 138, 141

radiation, from computers 67,
68
radon gas 75
recreational drugs 22, 72, 74
reflexology 105, 129, 149
reiki 110
relaxation 28, 29, 111
for sleeplessness 132–3
relaxation techniques 36–9
remedies and therapies
101–17
acupuncture 108–9
aromatherapy in 106
Bach flowers 117
chiropractic 102
homeopathy 114–15
hypnotherapy 111
medical herbalism 112–13
osteopathy 103
reflexology 105
reiki 110
shiatsu 116
Rhesus positive and negative
95
rubella (German measles) 24

safety belts, in cars 66
salmonella 53
salt 51, 123
sciatica 126
sex, during pregnancy 34
post-baby 35
timing for conception
24–5
shellfish, raw 50
shiatsu 116, 131
signals, basic body 31
skin problems 123
skincare products 82
sleeping 37, 121, 133
sleeplessness, remedies
132–3
smoking 22, 72, 73
special dietary needs 54–7
diabetic 56, 57
food intolerance and
allergies 56

vegetarian 54–6
spina bifida 97
spinach 44
sports, in pregnancy 28
stress levels 28–9
reducing 22–3, 68
stretch marks 123, 124
students 90
sugar, in pregnancy 51
swelling (edema) 124
swimming 27

tearing 90–1, 138, 145
TENS (Transcutaneous
Electrical Nerve
Stimulation) 147
tiredness 29, 121
toiletries 82
toxoplasmosis 53
Traditional Chinese Medicine
(TCM) 108
travel 66, 69
trimesters 14–19

ultrasound scans 93–4, 97
urinary tract infections
(cystitis) 128–9
uterus, after birth 139

vegetables 44, 50
vegetarian diet 54–6
visualization 37, 111
vitamin A 46, 47, 51
vitamin B6 59
vitamin C 46, 131
vitamin D 45, 59
vitamin E 46, 123, 124
vitamin K 91, 142
vitamins,
overdoses 46, 47
supplements 23

walking 27
wallpaper 77
watercress 44
weight, pre-conceptual 23
weight gain 62–3
work, during pregnancy 66–9

X-rays 75

yoga 27, 36–7, 126
yogurt 45

zinc 45, 124

Picture Credits

Key: l=left, r=right, c=center, t=top, b=bottom

p1 FANCY/Tammy Hanratty
p2 Loupe/Debi Treloar
p3 Loupe/Winfried Heinze
p5t Loupe/David Montgomery
p5c Loupe/Debi Treloar
p5b Loupe/Winfried Heinze
p6 Image Source
p9, 10 Loupe/Debi Treloar
p12–13 Cultura/Frank and Helena
p14 Anatomical Travelogue/Science Photo Library
p15tl/tc Anatomical Travelogue/Science Photo Library
p15tr Science Pictures Ltd/Science Photo Library
p15b Dr Najeeb Layyous/Science Photo Library
p16tl James Stevenson/Science Photo Library
p16tr Edelmann/Science Photo Library
p16bl Dr Najeeb Layyous/Science Photo Library
p16br Hank Morgan/Science Photo Library
p17tl Neil Bromhall/Science Photo Library
p17tr Chuck Swartzell, Visuals Unlimted.Science Photo Library
p17bl Gustoimages/Science Photo Library
p17br CIMN, ISM/Science Photo Library
p18tl Anatomical Travelogue/Science Photo Library
p18tc BSIP, ATL/Science Photo Library
p18tr Bernard Benoit/Kretz Technik/Science Photo Library
p18b Zephyr/Science Photo Library
p19t Edelmann/Science Photo Library
p19br Matt Meadows/Science Photo Library
p20 Getty Images/Jamie Grill
p23 Getty Images/Mimi Haddon
p25 Cultura/Brigitte Sporrer
p26 Loupe/Winfried Heinze
p27 Alamy/Moose Azim
p29 Loupe/Debi Treloar
p30 Cultura/Ghislain & Marie David de Lossy
p31 Loupe/Daniel Farmer

p33 Ojo Images/Paul Bradbury
p35t John Dowland
p35b Corbis
p36 Ian Hooton/Science Photo Library
p38 Image Source/Nigel Riches
p39 CICO Books/Geoff Dann
p42 Food Collection
p44 Aflo Ink/Nobuyuki Yoshikawa
p45 Glow Images/Cathy Yeulet
p46l Glow Images/Elena Elisseeva
p46r Loupe/Patrice de Villiers
p47 Glow Images/Elena Elisseeva
p48 Loupe/Richard Jung
p49 Loupe/Peter Cassidy
p50 Loupe/David Munns
p51 Loupe/Winfried Heinze
p52t Loupe/Nicki Dowey
p52b Getty Images/Tyler Edwards
p53t Loupe/David Montgomery
p53b Loupe/Francesca Yorke
p54 Loupe/Martin Brigdale
p55 Loupe/Debi Treloar
p57 Loupe/William Reavell
p59 Loupe/Debi Treloar
p60 Loupe/Richard Jung
p61 Loupe/Richard Jung
p63 Loupe/Dan Duchars
p64 Jupiter Images
p66 Rubberball/Mike Kemp
p67 Blend/JGI
p68 AsiaPix/Nugene Chiang
p70 Loupe/David Montgomery
p73 CICO Books/Mark Scott
p75 Corbis/Peter Reali
p76 Loupe/Debi Treloar
p77, 78 CICO Books/Christopher Drake
p81, 82, 83 Loupe/Winfried Heinze
p84, 87 Ian Hooton/Science Photo Library
p89 Loupe/Dan Duchars
p91 Ian Hooton/ Science Photo Library
p93 Tetra Images
p94 Superstock/Hill Creek Pictures
p95 Ian Hooton/Science Photo Library
p97 Stock Connection/Frank Chmura

p99 Blend/Jose Luis Pelaez Inc
p100 Getty Images/Ruth Jenkinson
p104, 107 CICO Books/Tino Tedaldi
p108 Glow Images/Yuri Arcurs
p109 Tetra Images/Yuri Arcurs
p110 Glow Images/Dean Mitchell
p111 Glow Images/Andres Rodriguez
p113t Loupe/David Montgomery
p113b Liu Yang/Redlink/Corbis
p115 Tetra Images
p117 Loupe/David Montgomery
p118 Loupe/Dan Duchars
p121 Loupe/Dan Duchars
p122 Loupe/Winfried Heinze
p123 Loupe/Lisa Cohen
p125 Juice Images
p127 Westend 61/Claudia Rehm
p128 Loupe/Lisa Linder
p129t Food Collection
p129b CICO Books/Tino Tedaldi
p130 Chris Rout/Alamy
p131l Loupe/Nicki Dowey
p131r Food Collection
p133 CICO Books/Tino Tedaldi
p134 Blend/LWA/Larry Williams
p137 Jose Luis Pelaez Inc Jose Luis Pelaez Inc Blend Images/Jose Luis Pelaez Inc
p139 Glow Images/Alena Yakusheva
p141 Loupe/Debi Treloar
p142 Cultura/Aurelie and Morgan David de Lossy
p144 Moodboard
p146 Alamy/BC photography
p147 Image Source
p149 CICO Books/Tino Tedaldi
p150 Getty Images/Andersen Ross
p151 Rubberball/Herman du Plessis
p152 I Love Images
p153 Blend/Terry Vine
p155 Ojo Images/Ashley Gill

With thanks to The Studio Partner for assistance with picture research.

Author's Acknowledgments

Firstly, I would like to thank Gillian Haslam and Cindy Richards at CICO Books for their support and enthusiasm for this project, and thanks to Liz Dean. Also, my thanks to Chelsey Fox, my friend and agent, for helping to make it happen.

As ever, my overwhelming thanks for their constant support and understanding go to my husband, Nick, and my two sons, Alex and George, with whom I enjoyed carefree, natural, and joyful pregnancies.